LGBTQIA+ Health in Aging Adults

Editors

MANUEL ESKILDSEN
CARL HENRY BURTON

CLINICS IN GERIATRIC MEDICINE

www.geriatric.theclinics.com

Consulting Editor
G. MICHAEL HARPER

May 2024 • Volume 40 • Number 2

ELSEVIER

1600 John F. Kennedy Boulevard • Suite 1800 • Philadelphia, Pennsylvania, 19103-2899

http://www.theclinics.com

CLINICS IN GERIATRIC MEDICINE Volume 40, Number 2
May 2024 ISSN 0749–0690, ISBN-13: 978-0-443-12957-5

Editor: Taylor Hayes
Developmental Editor: Anita Chamoli

Clinics in Geriatric Medicine (ISSN 0749-0690) is published quarterly by Elsevier Inc., 360 Park Avenue South, New York, NY 10010-1710. Months of issue are February, May, August, and November. Business and Editorial Offices: 1600 John F. Kennedy Blvd., Suite 1800, Philadelphia, PA 191023-2899. Periodicals postage paid at New York, NY, and additional mailing offices. Subscription prices are $321.00 per year (US individuals), $100.00 per year (US & Canadian student/resident), $340.00 per year (Canadian individuals), $457.00 per year (international individuals), and $195.00 per year (international student/resident). For institutional access pricing please contact Customer Service via the contact information below. Foreign air speed delivery is included in all *Clinics* subscription prices. All prices are subject to change without notice. POSTMASTER: Send address changes to *Clinics in Geriatric Medicine,* Elsevier Health Sciences Division, Subscription Customer Service, 3251 Riverport Lane, Maryland Heights, MO 63043. **Telephone: 1-800-654-2452 (U.S. and Canada); 314-447-8871 (outside U.S. and Canada). Fax: 314-447-8029. E-mail:** journalscustomerservice-usa@elsevier.com **(for print support) or** journalsonlinesupport-usa@elsevier.com **(for online support)**.

Reprints. For copies of 100 or more, of articles in this publication, please contact the Commercial Reprints Department, Elsevier Inc., 360 Park Avenue South, New York, New York 10010-1710. Tel.: 212-633-3874; Fax: 212-633-3820, E-mail: reprints@elsevier.com.

Clinics in Geriatric Medicine is covered in *MEDLINE/PubMed (Index Medicus), EMBASE/Excerpta Medica, Current Contents/Clinical Medicine (CC/CM), and the Cumulative Index to Nursing & Allied Health Literature*.

Contributors

CONSULTING EDITOR

G. MICHAEL HARPER, MD
Professor of Medicine, Geriatrics Department of Medicine, University of California, San Francisco, San Francisco, California, USA

EDITORS

MANUEL ESKILDSEN, MD, MPH
Clinical Professor, Department of Medicine, University of California, Los Angeles, Los Angeles, California, USA

CARL HENRY BURTON, MD
Hospitalist, Department of Internal Medicine, VA, University of California, Los Angeles, Los Angeles, California, USA

AUTHORS

SEAN R. CAHILL, PhD
Director of Health Policy Research, Fenway Institute, Boston, Massachusetts, USA

ROHIN A. AGGARWAL, MD, MPH
Physician, Department of Medicine, Johns Hopkins University School of Medicine, Baltimore, Maryland, USA

JILL BLUMENTHAL, MD
Associate Professor, Department of Medicine, University of California San Diego, San Diego, California, USA

JENNIFER L. CARNAHAN, MD, MPH, MA
Assistant Professor, Physician, Department of Medicine, Indiana University School of Medicine, Roudebush VA Medical Center, Indianapolis, Indiana, USA

WENDY J. CHEN, MD
Hospitalist and Geriatrician, Department of Medicine, Loyola University Medicine Center, Chicago, Illinois, USA; Internal Medicine, Geriatrician, ACP AGS WPATH USPATH

MICHAEL DANIELEWICZ, MD
Assistant Professor, Pride at the Jefferson Center for Healthy Aging, Division of Geriatric Medicine and Palliative Care, Department of Family and Community Medicine, Director, Thomas Jefferson University, Philadelphia, Pennsylvania, USA

ERICA JOY ERNEY, BSW, MSW, LCSW
The Permanente Medical Group, Kaiser Permanente Santa Clara Medical Center, Santa Clara, California, USA

CYNTHIA D. FIELDS, MD
Assistant Professor, Department of Psychiatry and Behavioral Sciences, Johns Hopkins University School of Medicine, Baltimore, Maryland, USA

ZIL GOLDSTEIN, MSN, RN, FNP
Associate Medical Director for TGNB Health, Callen-Lorde Community Health Center, PhD Student, CUNY School of Public Health and Health Policy, New York, New York, USA

ALEXANDER B. HARRIS, MPH, CPH
Clinical Research Manager, Callen-Lorde Community Health Center, New York, New York, USA

NOELLE MARIE JAVIER, MD
Associate Professor, Icahn School of Medicine at Mount Sinai, New York, New York, USA

AMY JUSTICE, MD, PhD
Long Professor of Medicine (General Medicine) and Professor of Public Health (Health Policy), Department of General Internal Medicine, Yale School of Medicine, Yale University, West Haven, Connecticut, USA

MAILE YOUNG KARRIS, MD
Associate Professor, Department of Medicine, University of California San Diego, San Diego, California, USA

EVIE KALMAR, MD, MS
Physician, San Francisco Veterans Administration, University of California, San Francisco, San Francisco of Veterans Affairs Health, San Francisco, California, USA

MEGAN LAU, MD
Resident Physician, Department of Medicine, University of California San Diego, San Diego, California, USA

JEFFREY MARIANO, MD
Clinical Assistant Professor, Department of Geriatrics and Palliative Medicine, AGSF, Southern California Permanente Medical Group, Bernard J Tyson Kaiser Permanente School of Medicine, Kaiser Permanente West Los Angeles, Los Angeles, California, USA

ROY NOY, MD
Geriatric Resident, Tel Aviv Sourasky Medical Center, Tel Aviv-Yafo, Israel

AL OGAWA, MD
Swedish Cherry Hill Family Medicine Residency, Seattle, Washington, USA

ANDREW C. PICKETT, MSEd, PhD
Assistant Professor, Department of Health and Wellness Design, Indiana University Bloomington, Bloomington, Indiana, USA

ANGELA D. PRIMBAS, MD
Clinical Instructor, Division of Geriatrics, Department of Medicine, UCLA David Geffen School of Medicine, University of California, Los Angeles, Los Angeles, California, USA

ASA E. RADIX, MD, PhD, MPH
Senior Director of Research and Education, Physician, Department of Medicine, Callen-Lorde Community Health Center; Associate Professor of Clinical Epidemiology, Department of Epidemiology, Mailman School of Public Health, Columbia University, Columbia University Mailman School of Public Health; Clinical Professor, Department of Medicine, NYU Grossman School of Medicine, New York, New York, USA

MARIAH L. ROBERTSON, MD, MPH
Assistant Professor of Medicine, Division of Geriatric Medicine and Gerontology, Department of Internal Medicine, Johns Hopkins School of Medicine, Baltimore, Maryland, USA

MATTHEW L. RUSSELL, MD, MSc
Instructor in Medicine, Massachusetts General Hospital, Harvard University, Boston, Massachusetts, USA

LOREN SCHECHTER, MD
Professor of Surgery and Urology, Rush University Medical Center, Rush University, Chicago, Illinois, USA

VINITA GIDVANI SHASTRI, MD, GRECC
Clinical Assistant Professor, VA Palo Alto Health Care System, Affiliated, Stanford School of Medicine, Palo Alto, California, USA

MARIA H. VAN ZUILEN, PhD
Associate Professor, Department of Medical Education, University of Miami Miller School of Medicine (R53), Miami, Florida, USA

Contents

Foreword: Individualizing Care for Lesbian, Gay, Bisexual, Transgender, Queer, Intersex, and Asexual+ Older Adults **xiii**

G. Michael Harper

Preface **xv**

Manuel Eskildsen and Carl Henry Burton

Affirming Care for LGBTQ+ Patients **211**

Noelle Marie Javier and Roy Noy

The lesbian, gay, bisexual, transgender, and queer(LGBTQ +) community is a marginalized minority group who continues to face and experience significant discrimination, prejudice, stigma, oppression, and abuse in various societal domains including health care. The older adult LGBTQ + community is an especially vulnerable group as they have unique minority stressors attributed to intersectional identities of age, ableism, ethnicity, and employment, among other factors. It is critical for health care providers to recognize and mitigate disproportionate care by engaging in strategies that promote inclusion and affirmation of their sexual orientation and gender identity. The biopsychosocial, cultural, and spiritual framework is a useful tool to care for this community in a holistic and compassionate way.

Preventive and Sexual Health in LGBTQ+ Older Adults **223**

Maile Young Karris, Megan Lau, and Jill Blumenthal

Sexual health is an important but often overlooked health concern of LGBTQ + older adults. Multiple factors influence sexual health including intersecting identities; adverse life events; coping mechanisms; and psychological, social, and physical health domains. Thus, the use of a culturally competent and comprehensive person-centered approach to sexual health is warranted. In this review, we discuss approaches to engaging LGBTQ + older adults to ensure they are able to achieve their sexual health priorities and prevent new human immunodeficiency virus infections. We also discuss doxycycline postexposure prophylaxis to prevent other sexually transmitted infections and the impact of chemsex.

Medical Issues Affecting Older Gay and Bisexual Men **239**

Michael Danielewicz

Older gay and bisexual men constitute diverse, sizable, and potentially vulnerable populations. They have and continue to face discrimination and stigma in multiple settings, including health care. Older gay and bisexual men report worse health, higher rates of alcohol and tobacco use, and higher HIV rates compared with their heterosexual counterparts. They have unique needs and experiences in multiple realms of health care including mental health, sexual health, and cancer screenings. Geriatric medicine physicians and providers can educate themselves on these unique needs and risks and take steps to provide inclusive, affirming care.

Medical Issues Affecting Older Lesbian and Bisexual Women 251

Angela D. Primbas and Al Ogawa

Lesbian and bisexual (LB) women are a growing and understudied population in the United States. LB women have unique histories and health experiences and encounter numerous resource and health care disparities that impact healthy aging. Despite LB population growth, little research has investigated the experiences of LB women separately from the broader lesbian, gay, bisexual, transgender, queer or questioning, or another diverse gender identity (LGBTQ+) community. The research that does exist largely focuses on the experiences of younger LB women. Nonetheless, there are unique care considerations providers can enact to improve clinical care and address lifetimes of disparities and discrimination.

Gender-Affirming Care for Older Transgender and Gender Diverse Adults 261

Asa E. Radix, Loren Schechter, Alexander B. Harris, and Zil Goldstein

In the United States, it is estimated that 0.3% of Americans aged 65 and older, or almost 172,000 individuals, identify as transgender. Aging comes with a unique set of challenges and experiences for this population, including health care disparities, mental health concerns, and social isolation. It is crucial for clinicians to use a patient-centered and trauma-informed care approach to address their specific needs and provide evidence-based quality health care, including preventive screenings, mental health support, and advocating for legal protections.

Primary Care and Health Care of Transgender and Gender-Diverse Older Adults 273

Wendy J. Chen and Asa E. Radix

Clinicians working with older transgender and gender-diverse (TGD) individuals need to acquire the necessary knowledge and skills to provide care that is high quality and culturally appropriate. This includes supporting patients in their exploration of gender and attainment of gender-affirming medical interventions. Clinicians should strive to create environments that are inclusive and safe, and that will facilitate health care access and build constructive provider-patient relationships. Clinicians should be aware of best practices, including that age-appropriate health screenings should be anatomy based, and ensure that TGD older adults on gender-affirming hormone therapy (GAHT) receive ongoing laboratory monitoring and physical assessments, including serum hormone levels and biomarkers. Older TGD adults underutilize advance care planning, and need individualized assessments that consider their unique family structures, social support, and financial situation. End-of-life care services should ensure that TGD individuals are treated with dignity and respect.

Human Immunodeficiency Virus in Older Adults 285

Matthew L. Russell and Amy Justice

As people with HIV live longer, they can experience increased incidence and earlier onset of chronic conditions and geriatric syndromes. Older people are also at substantially increased risk of delayed diagnosis and treatment for HIV. Increasing provider awareness of this is pivotal in

these assessments and tools with sample scripts to provide patient-centered and holistic palliative care.

Home-Based Care for Lesbian, Gay, Bisexual, Transgender, Queer or Questioning, or another diverse gender identity Older Adults **347**

Mariah L. Robertson

The home-based medicine ecosystem is rapidly expanding. With this expansion, it is increasingly important to understand the unique needs of homebound older adults. There is likely significant intersectionality across the lesbian, gay, bisexual, transgender, queer or questioning, or another diverse gender identity (LGBTQ+) older adult population and the homebound population. This article begins to outline some strategies and approaches to entering the home of LGBTQ+ older adults in inclusive and trauma-informed ways and encourages home-based care teams, organizations, and health systems to utilize existing resources created by the LGBTQ+ aging community to provide universal skills training for the workforce.

Federal and State Policy Issues Affecting Lesbian, Gay, Bisexual, Transgender, and Queer Older Adults **357**

Sean R. Cahill

Anti-lesbian, gay, bisexual, transgender, and queer (LGBTQ) + discrimination is widespread, harming the health of LGBTQ + people and constituting a barrier to care. This contributes to higher rates of poverty among LGBTQ + people, especially among people of color, and lower insurance coverage rates. The Affordable Care Act's expansion of insurance access has reduced uninsurance rates among LGBT people and people living with human immunodeficienc virus (HIV). Systemic improvements in culturally responsive health care have occurred over the past decade, including increased collection and use of sexual orientation and gender identity data to improve quality of care. As older LGBTQ + people enter elder service systems, reforms are needed to ensure equitable access.

CLINICS IN GERIATRIC MEDICINE

FORTHCOMING ISSUES

August 2024
Pressure Injuries & Chronic Wounds
Jeffrey M. Levine, *Editor*

November 2024
Hypertension
Mark Supiano and Eric Tuday, *Editors*

February 2025
Geriatric Anesthesia
Shamsuddin Akhtar, *Editor*

RECENT ISSUES

February 2024
Geriatric Dermatology Update
Nicole Burkemper, *Editor*

November 2023
Geriatric Emergency Care
Maura Kennedy and Shan W. Liu, *Editors*

August 2023
Palliative Care
Kimberly Angelia Curseen, *Editor*

ISSUES OF RELATED INTEREST

Medical Clinics
https://www.medical.theclinics.com/
Primary Care: Clinics in Office Practice
https://www.primarycare.theclinics.com/

Foreword
Individualizing Care for Lesbian, Gay, Bisexual, Transgender, Queer, Intersex, and Asexual+ Older Adults

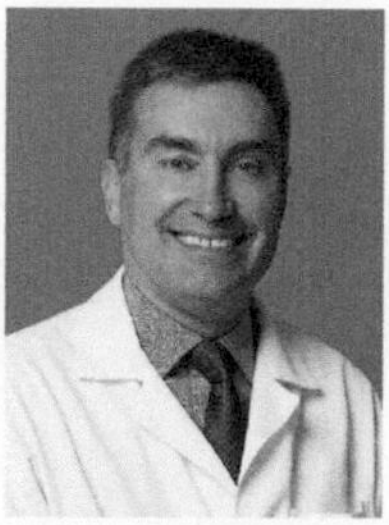

G. Michael Harper, MD
Consulting Editor

"If you've seen one 80-year-old, you've seen one 80-year-old." I can't remember exactly when I first heard this quote, but it has always resonated with me as a reminder of the importance to individualize care for older adults. It harkens to the heterogeneity of adults as they age. We often think about this type of heterogeneity in terms of age-related physiologic changes, but in the case of Lesbian, Gay, Bisexual, Transgender, Queer, Intersex, and Asexual+ (LGBTQIA)+ older adults, we also need to consider the lived experiences of members of this population. As our guest editors, Drs Manuel Eskildsen and Carl Henry Burton, describe, this growing portion of the older population has often felt and been invisible in the health care system. This invisibility, combined with decades of discrimination, has resulted in circumspection about the health care system and in health outcome disparities when compared with a population of heterosexual older adults.[1]

I have long thought of geriatrics health professionals as champions of the most vulnerable members of our communities, which is why I am so proud that *Clinics in Geriatric Medicine*, for the first time, is devoting an issue to LGBTQIA+ health in aging adults. This issue will cover wide-ranging topics that will help all clinicians improve their abilities to care for LGBTQIA+ older adults, care that acknowledges the unique barriers and challenges this group of individuals faces and affirms their value. There are articles that address primary care, preventive and sexual health, HIV, and mental health, while also tackling psychosocial and financial issues and federal and state policies that impact LGBTQIA+ older adults.

Clin Geriatr Med 40 (2024) xiii–xiv
https://doi.org/10.1016/j.cger.2024.02.001
0749-0690/24/Published by Elsevier Inc.

We all have the expectation of individualized care that respects our own unique background, experience, and health history. LGBTQIA+ older adults deserve the same. This issue is a leap in achieving that goal.

G. Michael Harper, MD
Geriatrics Department of Medicine
University of California, San Francisco
4150 Clement Street, Rm 310B
San Francisco, CA 94121, USA

E-mail address:
Michael.harper@ucsf.edu

REFERENCE

1. Fredriksen-Goldsen KI, Kim HJ, Barkan SE, et al. Health disparities among lesbian, gay, and bisexual older adults: results from a population-based study. Am J Public Health 2013;103(10):1802–9. https://doi.org/10.2105/AJPH.2012.301110. Epub 2013 Jun 13. PMID: 23763391.

Preface

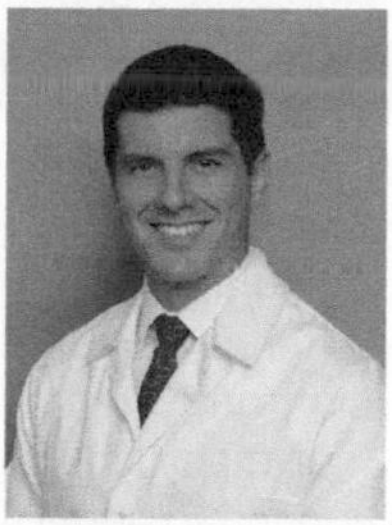
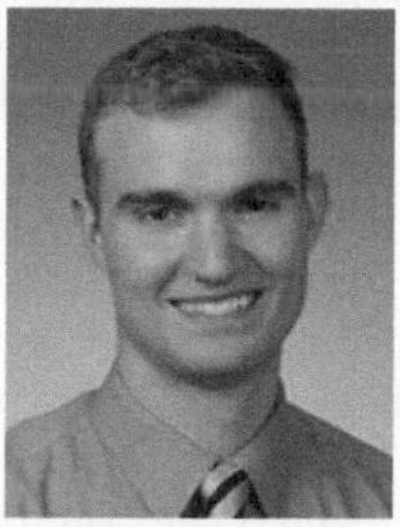

Manuel Eskildsen, MD, MPH Carl Henry Burton, MD
Editors

An estimated 2.7 million adults aged 50 years and older in the United States identify as lesbian, gay, bisexual, transgender, queer, or plus (LGBTQ+, also referred to sexual and gender minority [SGM]), which is expected to double by 2060 (please see Table 1, Chapter 1 for full definitions).[1] And of all adults, an estimated 7.2% identify as LGBT in 2022, with more older adults identifying as "gay."[2] Despite this growing number of LGBTQ+ older adults, they are often "invisible" within the health care system, facing a myriad of unique challenges informed by their past and present experiences.[3] For many, this invisibility was adaptive, as they would have faced discrimination and legal repercussions had they come out as LGBTQ+, even though paradoxically this hiding could further isolate community members and lead to stress and shame about the hidden identity.[4] Unfortunately, our legal system, society, and religious systems largely reinforced concealment LGBTQ+ identity for our many adults.[5] To understand how older LGBTQ+ members present to clinic, it is important to understand the intersection of their identity with experiences across the life span.

Discrimination against the LGBTQ+ community was the lifelong experience of many of LGBTQ+ older community members. This discrimination was written into law. Indeed, being gay was illegal in the lifetimes of many LGBTQ+ of an older generation. As recently as 1960, all US states had laws making same-sex sexual activity illegal. In over 10 states, this would last until a landmark ruling in 2003, *Lawrence v Texas*.[6,7] Consequently, many in today's LGBTQ+ older adult population lived with these injustices for the majority of their lives, with some enduring these conditions until just two decades ago. Beyond the criminalization of same-sex relations, there were compounded injustices, including housing discrimination, job bias, and the unjust removal of children from their parents. When examining these historical events, it's essential to understand the extensive challenges faced by LGBTQ+ older adults and how that impacts them to this very day, whether it be through internalized stigma or development of resiliency to better cope.

LGBTQ+ people were persecuted at various levels of society, including federal employment, reflective of widespread discrimination. One poignant example of this

Clin Geriatr Med 40 (2024) xv–xx
https://doi.org/10.1016/j.cger.2023.11.001

discrimination was the Lavender Scare of the late 1940s into the 1960s, where LGBTQ+ individuals were systematically persecuted based on nothing more than their sexual orientation or suspected orientation. Related to the Red Scare of McCarthyism, a presidential executive order sought to expel sexual minority federal employees based on their perceived threat to national security and "moral weakness." Thousands of employees were fired without justification or forced to resign as they were investigated for their sexuality. Beyond the immediate impact on the affected employees, the Lavender Scare had more far-reaching consequences. It cultivated a culture of fear and suspicion, where prospective employees would suppress or hide their LGBTQ+ identity to protect their careers and livelihoods. The fear even extended outside of the government, with LGBTQ+ individuals in Hollywood and New York City fearing they may be fired if their employer found out if they were gay. For many, the mere hint or suspicion of being a part of the LGBTQ+ community was enough to derail their professional aspirations.[8]

This period of intense discrimination came on the heels of a time when many LGBTQ+ individuals were starting to find solace and community in urban environments. Cities had become havens, where members of the community began to connect, form relationships, and establish their spaces. The Lavender Scare was in stark contrast to those strides toward finding space and was emblematic of the lack of tolerance, let alone equality, for LGBTQ+ people in the mid-twentieth century.[9]

The oppressive environment that the LGBTQ+ community endured for decades ultimately spurred increasingly assertive and bold advocacy. LGBTQ+ community resistance grew out of immense frustration from paradoxically having their existence ignored and persecuted. Throughout the 1960s, there were several police raids targeting LGBTQ+ spaces, which were met with increasing resistance from the community.[10] The Stonewall Uprising in June 1969 proved to be a watershed moment. The uprising was triggered by a police raid on the Stonewall Inn, a known gathering spot for LGBTQ+ people in Greenwich Village. Rather than accepting the raid as just another instance of harassment, the bar patrons, alongside neighborhood residents, resisted the police actions with unprecedented defiance.[11] The crowd quickly grew to over a hundred people, and eventually, thousands.[12]

Over the course of several days, these acts of resistance grew into larger demonstrations and confrontations with law enforcement. Importantly, the Stonewall Uprising was distinctive in its inclusivity, seeing significant diverse participation from drag queens, transgender people, and people of color.[13] Such diversity in advocacy underlined the broad scope of oppression the LGBTQ+ community faced and showcased the united front they presented against it.

The aftermath of the Stonewall Uprising was transformative as the LGBTQ+ community commemorated it. The Uprising gave rise to numerous gay rights organizations and directly led to the tradition of annual Pride Marches.[14] The legacy of Stonewall lives on in annual Pride Marches to this day. These yearly Pride festivities serve as a potent reminder of the struggle for LGBTQ+ rights, the progress made, and the journey ahead.[15]

In the health arena, LGBTQ+ adults were also experiencing discrimination as their gender and sexual identities were pathologized. In the early twentieth century, most psychiatrists regarded homosexuality as pathologic, and there were even attempts at psychoanalytic "cure."[16] In the first *Diagnostic and Statistical Manual of Mental Disorders* (*DSM*), homosexuality was not only pathologized but also perversely listed as a "sociopathic personality disturbance." This medical discrimination began changing, as there were increasing visibility and discussion of LGBTQ+ individuals, particularly in psychologist Alfred Kinsey's work. His 1948 and 1953 Kinsey reports included discussion of same-sex sexual desire and became best sellers, sparking discussion about the underrecognized and pathologized LGBTQ+ community. Moreover, Kinsey and his contemporaries revealed data that suggested homosexuality was not so rare, but likely an underrecognized, common identity.[17] This research, combined with activism after the Stonewall Riots, led to unprecedented educational panels from the gay community during annual American Psychiatric Association (APA) meetings in 1971 and 1972. The APA finally reevaluated the classification of homosexuality as a mental disorder, even evaluating what constitutes a mental disorder. Homosexuality was finally removed as mental illness from the *DSM* in 1973.[17]

For transgender and gender-diverse individuals, medical understanding took even longer. Kinsey and his contemporaries also spurred discussion about gender identity, at that time using the word "transexual" (a now outdated term) to describe transgender and gender-diverse individuals.[18] Unfortunately, for many practitioners, sexual orientation and gender identity were conflated, reflective of lack of understanding, and even less understanding of affirming care. Perhaps it was this lack of understanding that led to transgender and gender-diverse people being considered severely neurotic or psychotic, demonstrating severe pathologization of gender identity, by medical providers in the mid-twentieth century.[16]

Despite frank medical pathologization, some patients were able to find pioneering affirming care. The first transgender adult to publicly discuss their gender-affirming surgery was Christine Jorgensen in 1952, which led to greater awareness of gender identity.[16] During the 1960s and 1970s, there was expansion in understanding and care for transgender and gender-diverse patients. However, 1979 saw the closure of the gender identity clinic at Johns Hopkins, an unfortunate setback for the progress of providing gender-affirming care. During the 1980s and 1990s, Dr. Henry Benjamin established the World Professional Association for Transgender Health, and in response to earlier criticism on care for transgender people, developed the Standards of Care (SOC), providing guidelines for the medical treatment of transgender individuals.[18] The SOC provided guidance on gender-affirming care, including hormone therapy and surgical therapy, to better standardize gender-affirming care. However, being transgender was pathologized further when it was added to the *DSM* as "gender identity disorder" in 1980, a status that would not change until 2013.[18] When the *DSM* pathologized sexual and gender identity, it permitted discrimination and even contributed to harmful and inappropriate "conversion" or "reparative" therapies.[17] Removal of gender identity disorder from the *DSM* was an important step toward fair and just treatment of transgender and gender-diverse adults.

One of the most significant historical traumas impacting the LGBTQ+ community, especially transgender women and gay and bisexual men, was the HIV/AIDS epidemic in the 1980s and 1990s. The government's initial lack of response and the intense stigma associated with the disease resulted in significant loss and trauma within the community, though it also spurred community action and advocacy.[19] Today, many older gay and bisexual men are long-term survivors of HIV or have experienced significant loss due to AIDS, impacting their physical and mental health needs.[20]

The 1990s into the 2000s saw a large public change in visibility of LGBTQ+ people. With shows like "Will & Grace" featuring gay characters, to the sitcom "Ellen" featuring Ellen DeGeneres coming out of the closet as a lesbian on her sitcom, lesbian and gay people were suddenly visible. Even in politics, record numbers of LGBTQ+ people were serving as elected officials by the 2010s. Unfortunately, transgender and gender-diverse visibility was much later in the media, with 2014 bringing Laverne Cox as an openly transgender person to the cover of *Time* magazine.[21] Altogether, such visibility helped challenge preheld conceptions and stereotypes, humanizing

LGBTQ+ people.[22] It is thought that as a minority group, the pervasiveness of LGBTQ+ people, across every socioeconomic, ethnic, and even age group, meant that people knew LGBTQ+ people, which helped dispel discriminatory myths of LGBTQ+ identity, particularly LGB identity.

Ultimately, the legal recognition of same-sex marriage in 2015 by the Supreme Court's ruling in *Obergefell v Hodges* was a significant step toward equality. However, this relatively recent change means that many older LGBTQ+ adults spent most of their lives without the legal protections and benefits that marriage provides, such as spousal benefits and end-of-life decision-making rights. In addition, discriminatory policies, such as the Defense of Marriage Act of 1996, which was in effect until 2013, meant that same-sex couples were not recognized at the federal level, excluding them from federal benefits afforded to other married couples.[23]

Even though there has been great progress in LGBTQ+ equality, transgender and gender-diverse people remain an extremely vulnerable group facing anti-transgender sentiment, discrimination, and legal threats. At the beginning of 2023, there were over 150 bills targeting transgender and gender-diverse people. And there are still barriers for LGBTQ+ individuals in health care. Discrimination is still legal in many areas of life in numerous states, and religious exemption laws can allow health care providers to refuse to care for LGBTQ+ people based on moral or religious objections.[24] This policy can be particularly detrimental to the health of those in rural areas where alternative care providers may not be available. Even after a lifetime of discrimination for LGBTQ+ older adults, there are still ongoing advocacy efforts within the LGBTQ+ community to seek equality, even in medical care.

An understanding of shared history in the LGBTQ+ community informs caring for LGBTQ+ older adults. This knowledge can guide health care providers in delivering care with cultural humility. Moreover, shared understanding can help create a trauma-informed environment that acknowledges the historical traumas and systemic discrimination these individuals have experienced. Future health care policies must prioritize inclusivity and equity to meet the needs of the diverse aging population.

When we understand this history, we see that the age at which LGBTQ+ older adults interfaced with large events like the Stonewall Riots and the first Gay Pride Marches affects how they were socialized to society and health care. For older adults who lived when being gay or transgender was considered a mental disorder, they may have adapted by being invisible. For those younger older adults, especially the baby boomers, they may have received more affirming health care, encouraging them to be "out" as their authentic selves. In the end, these events have deeply shaped the LGBTQ+ community, and providers can still provide affirming, trauma informed care to all who enter the clinical space, understanding the intersectionality of identity in age and beyond. Older LGBTQ+ adults are not monolithic—they are diverse in identity. They are diverse in sexuality. They are diverse in gender. They are diverse in ethnicity. They are diverse in socioeconomic class. They are diverse in age. This diversity provides intersectionality to the identities of our older adults and a richness of lived experience.

We hope to help you provide quality care for this diverse community. This issue covers topics from the clinical approach to the care of the diverse members of the LGBTQ+ community, to practical approaches to HIV in the older adult, to the challenges of caring for LGBTQ+ adults in long-term care settings or who are receiving palliative care. We believe that this issue will serve as a practical guide to providing equitable and compassionate care for this historically marginalized population.

Manuel Eskildsen, MD, MPH
Department of Medicine
University of California, Los Angeles
10945 Le Conte Avenue #2339
Los Angeles, CA 90095, USA

Carl Henry Burton, MD
Department of Internal Medicine
Greater Los Angeles VA, USA

University of California, Los Angeles
10945 Le Conte Avenue #2339
Los Angeles, CA 90095, USA

E-mail addresses:
meskildsen@mednet.ucla.edu (M. Eskildsen)
carl.burton@va.gov (C.H. Burton)

REFERENCES

1. Fredriksen-Goldsen KI, Espinoza R. Time for transformation: public policy must change to achieve health equity for LGBT older adults. Generations 2014;38(4): 97–106.
2. Jones J. US LGBT identification steady at 7.2%. Gallup 2023. Available at: https://news.gallup.com/poll/470708/lgbt-identification-steady.aspx. Accessed August 1, 2023
3. Jablonski RA, Vance DE, Beattie E. The invisible elderly: lesbian, gay, bisexual, and transgender older adults. J Gerontol Nurs 2013;39(11):46–52. https://doi.org/10.3928/00989134-20130916-02.
4. Pachankis JE, Mahon CP, Jackson SD, et al. Sexual orientation concealment and mental health: a conceptual and meta-analytic review. Psychol Bull 2020;146(10): 831–71. https://doi.org/10.1037/bul0000271.
5. Foster AB, Brewster ME, Velez BL, et al. Footprints in the sand: personal, psychological, and relational profiles of religious, spiritual, and atheist LGB individuals. J Homosex 2017;64(4):466–87. https://doi.org/10.1080/00918369.2016.1191237.
6. Unfair and unjust practices harm LGBTQ+ people and drive health disparities. CDC; 2023. Available at: https://www.cdc.gov/tobacco/health-equity/lgbtq/unfair-and-unjust.html. Accessed August 1, 2023.
7. Gilkis KB. Lawrence v. Texas. Legal Information Insitute. Cornell Law School; 2018.
8. Haynes S. You've probably heard of the Red Scare, but the lesser-known, anti-gay 'Lavender Scare' is rarely taught in schools. Time; 2020. Available at: https://time.com/5922679/lavender-scare-history/. Accessed August 1, 2023.
9. Adkins J. "These People Are Frightened to Death." Congressional investigations and the Lavender Scare. Prologue Magazine. National Archives; 2016. Available at: https://www.archives.gov/publications/prologue/2016/summer/lavender.html. I Publisher: The National Archives. Accessed August 2, 2023.
10. Hegarty P, Rutherford A. Histories of psychology after Stonewall: introduction to the special issue. Am Psychol 2019;74(8):857–67. https://doi.org/10.1037/amp0000571.

11. Halkitis PN. The Stonewall riots, the AIDS epidemic, and the public's health. Am J Public Health 2019;109(6):851–2. https://doi.org/10.2105/ajph.2019.305079.
12. The L. Stonewall: 50 years of fighting for their lives. Lancet 2019;393(10190): 2469. https://doi.org/10.1016/s0140-6736(19)31405-9.
13. Broady K. In: Romer C, editor. The black and brown activists who started pride. Brookings; 2021. Available at: https://www.brookings.edu/articles/the-black-and-brown-activists-who-started-pride/. Accessed August 8, 2023.
14. Armstrong EA, Crage SM. Movements and memory: the making of the Stonewall myth. Am Sociol Rev 71(5):724–751. doi:https://doi.org/10.1177/000312240607100502.
15. LGBTQ Activism. Library of Congress. Available at: https://www.loc.gov/classroom-materials/united-states-history-primary-source-timeline/post-war-united-states-1945-1968/lgbtq-activism/ Part of Library of Congress Classroom Materials at the Library of Congress U.S. History Primary Source Timeline The Post War United States, 1945 to 1968, LGBTQ Activism. Accessed August 8, 2023.
16. Drescher J. Queer diagnoses parallels and contrasts in the history of homosexuality, gender variance, and the Diagnostic and Statistical Manual (DSM) review and recommendations prepared for the DSM-V Sexual and Gender Identity Disorders Work Group. Focus (Am Psychiatr Publ) 2020;18(3):308–35. https://doi.org/10.1176/appi.focus.18302.
17. Drescher J. Out of DSM: depathologizing homosexuality. Behav Sci (Basel) 2015; 5(4):565–75. https://doi.org/10.3390/bs5040565.
18. Khan FN. A history of transgender health care. Scientific American 2016. Available at: https://blogs.scientificamerican.com/guest-blog/a-history-of-transgender-health-care/. Accessed August 9, 2023.
19. Francis DP. Toward a comprehensive HIV prevention program for the CDC and the nation. JAMA 1992;268(11):1444–7.
20. Emlet CA. "You're awfully old to have this disease": experiences of stigma and ageism in adults 50 years and older living with HIV/AIDS. Gerontologist 2006; 46(6):781–90. https://doi.org/10.1093/geront/46.6.781.
21. Fischer M. Introduction: a transgender tipping point?. In: Terrorizing gender: transgender visibility and the surveillance practices of the U.S. security. State University of Nebraska Press; 2019. Available at: muse.jhu.edu/book/68116. Pages 1–28. Accessed August 9, 2023.
22. Schmidt S. Americans' views flipped on gay rights. How did minds change so quickly? Washington Post 2019. Available at: https://www.washingtonpost.com/local/social-issues/americans-views-flipped-on-gay-rights-how-did-minds-change-so-quickly/2019/06/07/ae256016-8720-11e9-98c1-e945ae5db8fb_story.html. Accessed August 9, 2023.
23. Perone AK. Health implications of the Supreme Court's Obergefell vs. Hodges marriage equality decision. LGBT Health 2015;2(3):196–9. https://doi.org/10.1089/lgbt.2015.0083.
24. Religious Exemption Laws. Movement Advancement Project; 2023. Available at: https://www.lgbtmap.org/img/maps/citations-religious-exemption.pdf. Accessed August 1, 2023.

Affirming Care for LGBTQ + Patients

Noelle Marie Javier, MD[a,*], Roy Noy, MD[b]

KEYWORDS

• LGBTQ • Sexual and gender minorities • Affirming care • Inclusive care • Healthcare

KEY POINTS

- The lesbian, gay, bisexual, transgender, and queer (LGBTQ +) community, also known as sexual and gender minorities, is a diverse population who has historically experienced discrimination, prejudice, marginalization, and abuse that have resulted in significant health care disparities including disproportionate physical and mental health outcomes.
- A fundamental approach to providing an inclusive and affirming care practice is to develop a multidimensional understanding of the LGBTQ + community through a biopsychosocial, cultural, and spiritual framework; mitigate any form of harmful bias; and engage in a consistent cultural humility training for all staff.
- Key strategies to demonstrate inclusive and affirming care for the LGBTQ + community include visible indicators of support in office and clinical spaces; protective policies denouncing any form of discrimination toward the community; inclusion of sexual orientation and gender identity in medical intake forms; and the provision of resources among others.

INTRODUCTION

The lesbian, gay, bisexual, transgender, and queer (LGBTQ +) community, also known as sexual and gender minority (SGM) community, continues to be a highly vulnerable group because of the widespread experience of discrimination, prejudice, oppression, and abuse over time. As a result, they have received disproportionate medical care due to ongoing structural and systemic barriers that have led to significant physical and mental health outcomes.[1]

OVERVIEW OF HEALTH DISPARITIES

In 2011, the National Academy of Medicine recognized the significant gaps in knowledge and research towards the LGBTQ + community.[2] Similarly in 2015, the American

[a] Icahn School of Medicine at Mount Sinai, One Gustave L. Levy Place, 1070, New York, NY 10029, USA; [b] Tel Aviv Sourasky Medical Center, 6 Weizmann Street, Tel Aviv 6423906, Israel
* Corresponding author. Mount Sinai Hospital, One Gustave L. Levy Place, 1070, New York, NY 10029.
E-mail address: noelle.javier@mssm.edu

Clin Geriatr Med 40 (2024) 211–221
https://doi.org/10.1016/j.cger.2023.11.002
geriatric.theclinics.com
0749-0690/24/

College of Physicians emphasized the need for research to address health disparities affecting this community.[3] These disparities encompass both physical and mental health outcomes. A few examples include studies showing higher prevalence rates of cardiovascular and certain types of cancers among SGM men and women.[4,5] Additionally, there are data showing a higher risk for Hispanic SGMs to be newly diagnosed with human immunodeficiency virus (HIV) infection.[6,7] There is evidence showing higher rates of sexual assault toward SGM women compared to heterosexual women in the army.[8] Regarding mental health, a large study in the transgender community revealed a 40% lifetime suicide attempt rate that is nearly 9 times higher than the general population.[9] In the National Surveys on Drug Use and Health, SGM people were more likely than their non-SGMs counterparts to have had a mental illness including depression, suicidal ideation, and suicide attempts. The rates of opioid misuse are greater among bisexual and lesbian women compared to straight women in the past year. Bisexual men were about twice as likely as straight men to have misused opioids in the past year.[10]

DISCUSSION

Cultural Humility Versus Competency

Older LGBTQ + adults are a highly vulnerable population who continue to face discrimination and prejudice in various health care settings. The undesirable physical and mental health outcomes result from long-standing oppressive practices that health care institutions have propagated. In some states, LGBTQ + older adults are designated as a population of greatest social need.[11] It is essential to acknowledge the injustices that this community has experienced over the years. One strategy is engaging in a cultural humility and competency training. *Cultural humility* pertains to the recognition of power imbalance between a healthcare provider and a marginalized patient. It is also described as a self-reflective, open-minded, egoless, and supportive approach that integrates self-appraisal and reflection in daily interactions leading to open and respectful dialogue.[12] *Cultural Competency* describes the knowledge and understanding of a person's culture and adapting one's approach to health care by incorporating cultural differences and nuances.[13] Furthermore, it may have the limitation of implying that cultural aspects of health care are finite and can be taught and mastered in a single fixed curriculum, not fully encapsulating the heterogeneity of identity.[14] There is evidence showing that healthcare providers receive minimal training in cultural competency for the LGBTQ + community.[15,16]

Another strategy to mitigate discrimination and prejudice is through an intentional culture shift in the belief system, attitudes, and practices of healthcare providers. Retaining outdated or preconceived beliefs and judgments may be fraught with potentially harmful biases and prejudices that could lead to further stigmatization. Herek differentiates stigma based on sexual orientation, termed "sexual stigma," and that based on gender identity, referred to as "gender minority stigma."[17] Structural gender minority stigma leads to invisibility by preventing people from disclosing their gender identity when warranted such as in healthcare settings. Negative biases or stigma may wrongly label LGBTQ + identities as problematic, abnormal, inferior, and unnatural, particularly considering the pathologization of LGBTQ + identity by healthcare systems in the past, let alone legally and socially. Stigma manifests in various ways: it can be enacted, as seen in explicit abuse; perceived, which may lead individuals to live in stealth or remain closeted for fear of overt discrimination; or internalized, where individuals might experience self-loathing or guilt for being LGBTQ+ (such as internalized homophobia or homonegativity).[17] Moreover, these belief systems maybe grounded in cisgenderism and heterosexism. Given the implicit nature of these biases, unconscious bias training maybe a mitigating strategy.[18]

GUIDING PRINCIPLES AND CONSTRUCTS IN UNDERSTANDING AND ACKNOWLEDGING THE LGBTQ + COMMUNITY

In shaping the cultural lens of understanding toward the LGBTQ + community, there are some guiding principles worth practicing. Firstly, acknowledging sexual orientation and gender identity (SOGI) is a fundamental approach for inclusive and affirming care. *Sexual Orientation* is defined as a person's romantic, emotional, and sexual attraction to a gender or genders while *Gender Identity* refers to a person's internal sense or core of, being a man, woman, both, or neither.[19] Examples of SOGI are reflected in **Table 1**. In a 2017 study, the majority of respondents wanted providers to ask about their SOGI. While only 10% of patients reported not disclosing SOGI, more than two-thirds of the providers assumed that patients will refuse SOGI disclosure.[20] In a parallel study specifically looking at transgender patients, nearly 90% felt that sexual orientation was more important to disclose than gender identity. Nonetheless, the majority of the respondents reported that as long as SOGI was medically relevant, they were willing to disclose it.[21]

Secondly, it is also essential to understand that significant health outcomes are grounded in unique internal and external stressors. Ilan Meyer' *Minority Stress Model* underscores the importance of these stressors impacting the LGBTQ + community.[27] This framework illustrates that the LGBTQ + community may simultaneously experience additional stressors based on their SOGI while existing in society. The cumulative effect can become chronic and pervasive. These could lead to depression and anxiety. The model also describes proximal (internal) and distal stressors (external). Examples of proximal stressors include internalized homophobia or transphobia, and examples of distal stressors include hate crimes. Complementary to this construct is *allostatic load* that pertains to the aggregate burden of chronic stress and life events affecting a person(s).[28] When allostatic load exceeds the coping threshold, this will result in poorer health outcomes. As health care providers, we should be mindful of not only disparities in our patients, but also ways to support them in facing stress.

Thirdly, the constructs of *lived experiences* and *intersectionality* are important. The former recognizes that the LGBTQ + community has unique stories to tell and how important milestones and transition points have impacted and shaped them.[29] It may be governed by 2 theories. The *Life Course Theory* describes how older adults age over time and presupposes that a series of transitions and choice points are influenced both by the immediate social context, socio-historical period, and gender and social roles.[30] *Goal-oriented theories* regard adulthood and late-life development as a balance between gains and losses, pursuit of goals, and the development and maintenance of self.[31] On the other hand, *Intersectionality* pertains to the combination and intersection of internal and external factors and identities that affect, define, and shape the individual as a person.[32] Examples of these factors which may be equal or of variable degrees include class, language, ability, sexual orientation, gender identity, education, employment, religion, race, and other identities. The more minority identities a person has, the greater the likelihood of potential oppression and discrimination. That said, the LGBTQ + community has developed resources to be resilient. *Resilience* is defined as a set of learned behaviors and interpersonal relationships that precedes one's ability to cope with adversity. When specific efforts and adaptive behaviors are enacted, those are translated into coping efforts and buffering strategies.[33]

Table 1
Definitions of commonly used terms[22–26]

Term	Definition
Sexual orientation (SO)	A person's sexual, emotional, and relational attraction to specific gender(s). Examples include heterosexual, lesbian, gay, bisexual, pansexual, asexual, etc.
Gender identity (GI)	A person's internal sense of belonging or not to a specific gender. Examples: cisgender and transgender woman, cisgender and transgender man, non-binary, etc.
Sex assigned at birth (SAB)	A person's sex assignment at birth reflected on the birth certificate and based on the appearance of the external genitalia and chromosomes. Examples: male, female, intersex, other
Gender expression	The outward expression of personality, appearance, and behavior that are usually socio-culturally defined as feminine or masculine
Lesbian	Refers to a woman with emotional, romantic, or sexual attraction to other women
Gay	Refers to a person with emotional, romantic, or sexual attraction to people of the same gender
Bisexual	Refers to a person with physical, sexual, emotional, romantic attraction to both men and women. The attraction does not have to be divided equally between genders and at all times.
Transgender	A term that encompasses individuals whose gender identities diverge from the biological sex they were assigned at birth. Example: a transgender woman is assigned male sex at birth but identifies as a woman.
Gender non-conforming (GNC) or gender non-binary (GNB)	A person with a non-traditional gender expression or a person who identifies outside of the gender binary (man or woman).
Queer	A term that could be catch-all to describe people who do not identify exclusively as 1 SOGI. In the past, this was used as a derogatory term.
Questioning	People who are examining their SOGI.
Intersex	Describes people who at birth had sex traits of more than 1 gender. They are born with differences in sexual development in their external or internal genitalia, chromosomal makeup, and hormonal production and/or response. They are also described as People born with differences in sexual development (DSD).
Asexual	Describes people who do not experience, completely or partially, sexual attraction, desire, and practice toward others.
Cisgender/Cis	A person whose sex at birth aligns with their gender identity. Example: a person assigned female at birth and identifies as a woman.

(*continued on next page*)

Table 1
(continued)

Term	Definition
Pansexual/Pan	Describes people who can be attracted physically, sexually, emotionally, or spiritually to members of all genders.
Two-spirit	Replaced the term "berdache." Used as a pan-Indian term by some Native American communities to describe people who present both female and male traits (temperament, dress, lifestyle, work, and social role).
Plus (+)	The plus sign recognizes the varieties of SOGI.

Robustness pertains to the individual's ability to withstand external forces and stressors. Examples of resources for resiliency and robustness include intrapersonal strengths, family support, community connections, spirituality, and other social justice advocacies that allow them to bounce back and continue to thrive in society.[34,35] As providers, promoting robustness and resiliency can be a key part of caring for those who have faced oppression and discrimination.

MULTIDIMENSIONAL APPROACH FOR INCLUSIVE AND AFFIRMING CARE

Engel's biopsychosocial approach to pain is the inspiration for multidimensional and holistic care.[36] This has been adapted and extrapolated for practice in various subspecialties including geriatrics and palliative care. A proposed modification of this paradigm would be to include the spiritual and cultural aspects to comprehensive patient assessments.[37] (**Fig. 1**).

The biological aspect considers some of the known physical health disparities and outcomes that affect this population. Examples of relevant literature include evidence showing that SGM minority women and men are more prone to obesity,

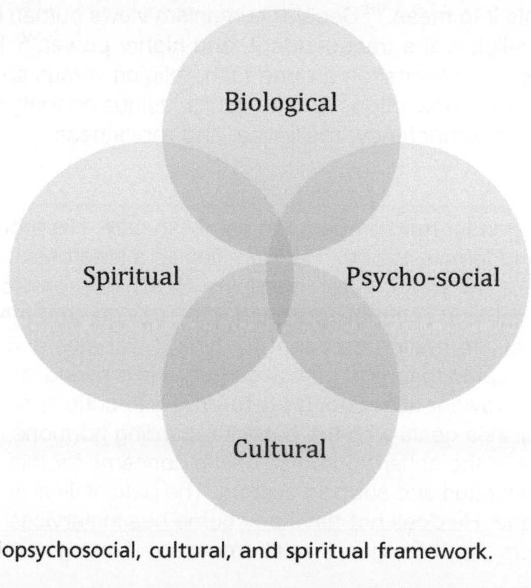

Fig. 1. Proposed biopsychosocial, cultural, and spiritual framework.

cardiovascular disease, neoplasms, hypertension, diabetes, and physical disability[38–40] Moreover, there are data showing that gay and bisexual men as well as transgender women have higher rates of human immunodeficiency virus (HIV) infection.[41] It is recommended that when a provider assesses the biological domain, the elements should include SOGI and comprehensive past and present medical histories including medication use.

The psychosocial aspect considers both mental health and psychosocial stressors. Experiences of victimization and abuse are associated with negative mental health and higher rates of lifetime suicide attempts.[42] Gay and bisexual men are observed to have higher rates of alcohol abuse, suicidal ideation, and internalized homophobia compared to gay and bisexual women.[42,43] There is evidence that a third of older SGM adults reported depressive symptoms and internalized ageism.[44] The National Transgender Discrimination Survey showed that the rate of lifetime suicide attempts for this population reached 41%. This sobering data should prompt clinicians including social workers to be attentive to the patient's lived experiences, mental health, minority stressors, crisis competency, resources for resilience and robustness, disenfranchised grief, and social supports including families of choice.[45]

The cultural aspect requires healthcare providers to be respectfully curious about the beliefs, values, and practices of the LGBTQ + patients and their families. It is important to recognize the diversity within the community. Be cognizant of the inadvertent practice of *Ethnocentrism* which is defined as the tendency to feel that one's own cultural norms are correct and superior while evaluating other's beliefs in light of them.[46] The elements in a cultural context include SOGI disclosure, lived experiences, unique minority stressors, biases, and resources for resiliency and robustness.

Finally, the spiritual aspect considers religion and spirituality, important considerations in understanding the full identity of our patients. *Religion* is characterized by institutional beliefs, practices, and rituals and while *Spirituality* may overlap, spirituality is an individualized journey influenced by experiential domains such as transcendence, connectedness, meaning, purpose, and energy among others.[47] Religion is often organized as a community but can also exist outside of an institution and may be practiced in private. In contrast, spirituality is broadly self-defined and can be anything a person wants it to mean.[46] Secular humanism views human existence without reference to God, religion, the transcendent, and higher power.[48] The elements in a spiritual context include information around faith, religion versus spirituality, intrapersonal and interpersonal connections and supports, unique minority stressors, and resources around crisis competency, resilience, and robustness.

Case Study

A 75-year-old transgender man presents to establish care. His pronouns are he/him/his. He was assigned female at birth. He identifies as a heterosexual man and brings along his spouse of 19 years. After obtaining SOGI, the provider uses the biopsychosocial, cultural, and spiritual approach. The provider and the interprofessional team gather medical information pertinent for type 2 diabetes and hypertension. He had top surgery and opted to forego genital surgery. He is taking intramuscular testosterone weekly. The provider assesses drug-to-drug interactions and adverse effects. The provider establishes goals with the patient regarding hormone replacement therapy . The provider and the patient prioritize health concerns for this visit. The provider explores his living situation and support system. The patient lives in an elevator apartment. He uses a cane. He does not have any home health services. He has two adult children with whom he has good relations with. Throughout his life, he has experienced discrimination. The social worker utilizes a trauma-informed approach in exploring minority stressors and lived experiences. He was disowned by his family and worked hard to finance his education. He managed to finish marketing and retired 10 years ago. He identifies as spiritual. He is active at the local senior center. He volunteered during the height of the HIV-acquired immunodeficiency syndrome (AIDS) epidemic. The provider assists him in filling out a healthcare proxy form. The provider offers a referral to chaplaincy and spiritual support. The social worker provides resources such as home services and support group referral. The provider proceeds to do a physical examination after asking permission. A summary of the comprehensive geriatric plan was discussed with the patient and his spouse with close follow-up in a month. This case illustrates the interprofessional team-based approach in providing affirming and inclusive care utilizing the biopsychosocial, spiritual, and cultural framework. Interventions utilized included appropriate use of SOGI; inclusion of the spouse; comprehensive evaluation integrating trauma-informed care and including the minority stressors, intersectionality, resiliency, and lived experiences; optimal use of resources; and close follow-up and collaboration among others.

SUMMARY

The LGBTQ + community is a highly vulnerable and marginalized group that has experienced and continues to face ongoing discrimination, prejudice, abuse, and oppression. This has resulted in undesirable physical and mental health outcomes. An intentional culture shift in the mindset, training, research, and practices in diverse clinical spaces is paramount to providing high-quality geriatric care. Having a fundamental understanding of core constructs impacting the LGBTQ + community is a good initial step in an ongoing cultural humility and competency training. A multidimensional approach to care using the proposed biopsychosocial, cultural, and spiritual framework may be an effective strategy to address unique needs and concerns. Some concrete examples of inclusive and affirming care include SOGI collection, visible indicators of support for the community, availability of resources, hiring LGBTQ + staff, and enforcing protective policies for the LGBTQ + community.

CLINICS CARE POINTS: PRACTICAL RECOMMENDATIONS FOR INCLUSIVE AND AFFIRMING MEDICAL CARE

The following are concrete strategies to provide an inclusive and affirming space to the LGBTQ + community.

1. Ensure that visible indicators for diverse patients are seen in various settings. These include welcoming signs, rainbow flags, gender-neutral bathrooms, pronoun pins, magazines, etc. A readable non-discrimination statement provides a safe space for the LGBTQ + community.[49] Moreover, hiring LGBTQ + staff will further reinforce this affirming setting.
2. SOGI should be integrated in the electronic records as part of the demographic information. A question around sex assigned at birth and pronouns should be included as well.[50]
3. For clinicians, review the medical chart beforehand and if SOGI is disclosed, to properly address the individual by name and pronouns. Introduce yourself with your name and pronouns. If SOGI has not been obtained, ask during the clinical encounter. Additionally, if the patient is not comfortable in disclosing SOGI, reassure that this could be deferred for now. Having an opt-out mechanism for SOGI disclosure may assist in alleviating any discomfort. Examples of SOGI questions: What are your pronouns? How would you

describe your sexual orientation? What is your gender identity? What was the sex assigned to you at birth or on your birth certificate?

4. If members of the patient's chosen and/or nuclear families are around, offer an invitation (with the patient's permission) to join the clinical encounter. This signals that as a provider you recognize the network of support.
5. During the clinical encounter, allow the patient to tell their story. Have them take the lead in how much information they would like to share. A good icebreaker question is Chochinov's Dignity Question: *"What do I need to know about you as a person to give you the best care possible?"*[51]
6. During history taking, de-stigmatizing language matters. Normalize conversations around sexual and reproductive health. Examples of inclusive and affirming language: Who are the important people in your life? What is your relationship status? Which gender identities are you attracted to? For transgender and gender diverse individuals, being mindful of potentially intrusive questions can foster trust. Examples include questions about genitalia and types of affirming treatments when not relevant to the chief concern; using deadnames (their names on their legal document such as birth certificates); using the wrong pronouns; and giving unwanted compliments.
7. Mirror patient language. If someone refers to their partner as their "roommate," which may occur in older adults, use this language (while clarifying what it means to them). For body parts for transgender and gender diverse people, it can also be affirming to refer to their body parts using their self-defined terms.
8. When mistakes occur (such as misgendering), apologize and move on. Mistakes do happen, so it is important to approach these situations with humility and not belabor your own mistake, but to instead learn from them for future patient care.
9. Ask permission and explain the rationale for a physical examination. Allow the patient to take the lead in which body parts are appropriate to be examined. Do a full anatomic inventory (with permission and explanation) for transgender and gender diverse patients since not everyone will have gender affirming surgeries. This will be especially relevant during annual wellness physical examinations and health maintenance screenings and will often be less relevant in some urgent care and follow-up visits.[52]
10. When doing a comprehensive geriatric assessment, integrating the biopsychosical, cultural, and spiritual framework will be a helpful tool for a holistic and multidimensional approach by integrating minority stressors, intersectionality, lived experiences, unconscious bias, SOGI, and resiliency. Having an interprofessional team working with patients and families is paramount.[53]
11. Part of a comprehensive geriatric assessment is advance care planning discussions. This includes completion of a living will and a health care proxy.[53,54]
12. It is recommended to have a repository of LGBTQ + resources for patients, families, and staff. Examples include access to Fenway Health, Callen Lorde, Services and Advocacy for GLBT Elders (SAGE), Human Rights Campaign (HRC), University of California in San Francisco (UCSF) Transgender Care, National Resource Center on LGBT Aging, etc.
13. An empowering practice for advocacy and safety is ensuring that protective, non-oppressive policies are in place to avoid any form of bias, discrimination, and abuse. An example would be respect for patient bill of rights regardless of SOGI and the presence of non-discrimination statements visible in the clinical and non-clinical spaces. An intentional and thoughtful cultural shift in the workplace can positively impact this community.[53,54]
14. Equally important is the allocation of resources and investment in research around gaps in care for the LGBTQ + community.[53,54]
15. When you witness a microaggression against LGBTQ + folks, silence is not a neutral response. Speak up and address issues that arise. Advocate for fair and just treatment of all individuals in your clinic.

DISCLOSURE

We do not have any financial disclosures.

REFERENCES

1. Javier NM, Oswald AG. Health for the lesbian, gay, bisexual, transgender, and queer (LGBTQ) older adults. Curr Geri Rep 2019;8:107–16.
2. Institute of Medicine. The health of Lesbian, Gay, Bisexual, and Transgender people: Building a Foundation for Better Understanding. Washington, DC: The National Academies Press, 2011. Available at: https://www.ncbi.nlm.nih.gov/books/NBK64806/pdf/Bookshelf_NBK64806.pdf. Accessed Aug 30, 2023.
3. Daniel H, Butkus R. Health and public policy committee of American College of Physicians. Lesbian, gay, bisexual, and transgender health disparities: executive summary of a policy position paper from the American College of Physicians. Ann Intern Med 2015 Jul 21;163(2):135–7.
4. Jackson CL, Agénor M, Johnson DA, et al. Sexual orientation identity disparities in health behaviors, outcomes, and services use among men and women in the United States: a cross-sectional study. BMC Publ Health 2016 Aug 17;16(1):807.
5. Saunders CL, Meads C, Abel GA, et al. Associations between sexual orientation and overall and site-specific diagnosis of cancer: evidence from two National patient Surveys in england. J Clin Oncol 2017 Nov 10;35(32):3654–61.
6. HIV Surveillance Report, 2021. Centers for Disease Control and Prevention website.Last update May 23,2023. Available at: http://www.cdc.gov/hiv/library/reports/hiv-surveillance.html. Accessed August 28, 2023.
7. Sullivan PS, Satcher-Johnson A, Pembleton ES, et al. Epidemiology of HIV in the USA: epidemic burden, inequities, contexts, and responses. Lancet 2021; 397(10279):1095–106.
8. Mattocks KM, Sadler A, Yano EM, et al. Sexual victimization, health status, and VA healthcare utilization among lesbian and bisexual OEF/OIF veterans. J Gen Intern Med 2013;28(Suppl 2):604–8.
9. James SE, Herman JL, Rankin S, Keisling M, Mottet L, Anafi M. The Report of the 2015 U.S. Transgender Survey. Washington, DC: National Center for Transgender Equality. Published 2016. Available at: http://www.ustranssurvey.org/reports#USTS. Accessed August 28, 2023.
10. Substance Abuse and Mental Health Services Administration. 2023. Lesbian, gay, and bisexual behavioral health: Results from the 2021 and 2022 National Surveys on Drug Use and Health (SAMHSA Publication No. PEP23-07-01-001). Center for Behavioral Health Statistics and Quality, Substance Abuse and Mental Health Services Administration. Available at: https://www.samhsa.gov/data/report/LGB-Behavioral-Health-Report-2021-2022 .Accessed August 28, 2023.
11. Available at: https://www.sageusa.org/wp-content/uploads/2023/07/sage-annual-report-2022-1.pdf. Accessed August 28, 2023.
12. Foronda C, Baptiste DL, Reinholdt MM, et al. Cultural humility: a concept analysis. J Transcult Nurs 2016;27:210–7.
13. Stubbe DE. Practicing cultural competence and humility in the care of diverse patients. Focus 2020;18(1):49–51.
14. Tervalon M, Murray-Garcia J. Cultural humility versus cultural competence: a critical distinction in defining physician training outcomes in multicultural education. J Health Care Poor Underserved 1998;9(2):117–25.

15. Obedin-Maliver J, Goldsmith ES, Stewart L, et al. Lesbian, gay, bisexual, and transgender-related content in undergraduate medical education. JAMA 2011; 306:971–7.
16. Dorsen C. An integrative review of nurse attitudes towards lesbian, gay, bisexual, and transgender patients. Can J Nurs Res 2012;44:18–43.
17. Herek GM. A nuanced view of stigma for understanding and addressing sexual and gender minority health disparities. LGBT Health 2016;3(6):397–9.
18. Available at: file:///Users/noeljavi/Downloads/learning-to-address-implicit-bias-towards-lgbtq-patients-case-scenarios.pdf. Accessed August 28, 2023.
19. Available at: https://eca.state.gov/files/bureau/sogi_terminology.pdf. Accessed August 28, 2023.
20. Haider AH, Schneider EB, Kodadek LM, et al. Emergency department query for patient-centered approaches to sexual orientation and gender identity: the Equality Study. JAMA Intern Med 2017;177(6):819–28.
21. Maragh-Bass AC, Torain M, Adler R, et al. Is it okay to ask: transgender patient perspectives on sexual orientation and gender identity collection in healthcare. Acad Emerg Med 2017;24:1–13.
22. Glossary of terms. Human Rights Campaign website. Available at: https://www.hrc.org/resources/glossary-of-terms. Accessed August 28, 2023.
23. Understanding the Health Needs of LGBT People. National LGBT Health Education Center. Available at: https://www.lgbtqiahealtheducation.org/wp-content/uploads/LGBTHealthDisparitiesMar2016.pdf. Accessed August 28, 2023.
24. Terminology Resource. National LGBT Cancer Network. Available at: https://cancer-network.org/resources/lgbt-terminology-resource/?gclid=CjwKCAjwxOymBhAFEiwAnodBLFfUJ-lWZaqL0J3Dwt3LtaOdYsQo6qM5x_L2_T_7-HRFPww6JZNMmhoCEIwQAvD_BwE. Accessed August 28, 2023.
25. Two-Spirit. Indian Health Service. Available at: https://www.ihs.gov/lgbt/health/twospirit/. Accessed August 28, 2023.
26. Available at: https://medicine.yale.edu/lgbtqi/curriculum/2021-07-04-lgbtqia_glossary_417482_37430_v3.pdf. Accessed August 29, 2023.
27. Meyer IH. Prejudice, social stress, and mental health in lesbian, gay, and bisexual populations: conceptual issues and research evidence. Psychol Bull 2003; 129(5):674–97.
28. Guidi J, Lucente M, Sonino N, et al. Psychother Psychosom 2021;90:11–27.
29. https://www.ncbi.nlm.nih.gov/pmc/articles/PMC8642108/. Accessed August 28, 2023.
30. Aldwin CM, Igarashi H, Gilmer DF, et al. Health, illness, and optimal aging: biological and psychological perspectives. 2nd edition. New York: Springer Publishing Company; 2013.
31. Van Wagenen A, Driskell J, Bradford J. I'm still raring to go: successful aging among lesbian, gay, bisexual, and transgender older adults. J Aging Stud 2013;27:1–14.
32. Seng J, Lopez W, Sperlich M, et al. Marginalized identities, discriminate burden and mental health: empirical exploration of an interpersonal-level approach to modeling intersectionality. Soc Sci Med 2012;75:2437–45.
33. Meyer IH. Resilience in the study of minority stress and health of sexual and gender minorities. Psychol Sex Orient Gender Divers 2015;2:209–13.
34. Smith MS, Gray SW. The courage to challenge: a new measure of hardiness in LGBT adults. J Gay Lesbian Soc Serv 2009;21:73–89.
35. Colpitts E, Gahagan J. The utility of resilience as a conceptual framework for understanding and measuring LGBTQ health. Int J Equity Health 2016;15:60.

36. Borrell-Carrio F, Suchman AL, Epstein RN. The biopsychosocial model 25 years later: principles, practice, and scientific inquiry. Ann Fam Med 2004;2(6):576–82.
37. Oh B, Klein P, Rosenthal DS, et al. Are we ready for a true biopsychosocial-spiritual model? The many meanings of "spiritual". Medicines (Basel) 2017; 4(4):79.
38. Wallace S, Cochran S, Durazo E, et al. The health of aging lesbian, gay, and bisexual adults in California. Los Angeles: UCLA Center for Health Policy Research; 2011.
39. Fredriksen-Goldsen KI, Kim HJ, Barkan SE, et al. Health disparities among lesbian, gay, and bisexual older adults: results from a population-based study. Am J Publ Health 2013;103(10):1802–9.
40. Fredriksen-Goldsen KI. Resilience and disparities among lesbian, gay, bisexual, and transgender older adults. Public Policy Aging Report 2011;21(3):3–7.
41. Yarns BC, Abrams JM, Meeks TW, et al. The mental health of older LGBT adults. Curr Psychiatr Rep 2016;18(60):1–11.
42. Cahill S, Singal R, Grasso C, et al. Do ask, Do tell: high levels of acceptability by patients routine collection of sexual orientation and gender identity data in four diverse American community health centers. PLoS One 2014;9(9):1–8.
43. Choi SK, Meyer IL. LGBT aging: a review of research findings, needs, and policy implications. The Williams Institute, UCLA School of Law; 2016.
44. Carter PL, Reardon SF. Inequality matters. New York: William T. Grant Foundation; 2014 Septmeber. https://wtgrantfoundation.org/library/uploads/2015/09/Inequality-Matters.pdf. Accessed August 29, 2023.
45. http://transexualia.org/wp-content/uploads/2015/03/Sanidad_ntdsreportonhealth.pdf. Accessed August 29, 2023.
46. Van der Geest S. How social science and medicine relate and should relate to one another. Soc Sci Med 1995;40(7):869–72.
47. Pesut B, Fowler M, Taylor EJ, et al. Conceptualising spirituality and religion for healthcare. J Clin Nurs 2008;17:2803–10.
48. Koenig HG. Religion, spirituality, and health: a review and update. Adv Mind Body Med 2015;29(3):19–26.
49. Coren JS, Coren CM, Pagliaro SN, et al. Assessing your office for care of lesbian, gay, bisexual, and transgender patients. Health Care Manag 2011;30(1):66–70.
50. Rullo JE, Foxen JL, Griffin JM, et al. Patient acceptance of sexual orientation and gender identity questions on intake forms in outpatient clinics: a pragmatic randomized multisite trial. Health Serv Res 2018;53(5):3790–808.
51. Chochinov HM, McClement S, Hack T, et al. Eliciting personhood within clinical practice: effects on patients, families, and health care providers. J Pain Symptom Manag 2015;49(6):974–80.
52. Bhatt N, Cannella J, Gentile JP. Gender-affirming care for transgender patients. Innov Clin Neurosci 2022;19(4–6):23–32.
53. Fredriksen-Goldsen KI, Hoy-Ellis CP, Goldsen J, et al. Creating a vision for the future: key competencies and strategies for culturally competent practice with lesbian, gay, bisexual, and transgender (LGBT) older adults in the health and human services. J Gerontol Soc Work 2014;570(0):80–107.
54. Javier NM. Palliative care needs, concerns, and affirmative strategies for the LGBTQ population. Palliat Care Soc Pract 2021;9:15.

Preventive and Sexual Health in LGBTQ+ Older Adults

Maile Young Karris, MD*, Megan Lau, MD, Jill Blumenthal, MD

KEYWORDS

- STI prevention • Sexual health screening • LGBTQ older adult • HIV PrEP
- Intersectionality

KEY POINTS

- Sexual health is an important component of well-being for LGBTQ + older adults.
- A culturally competent sexual history fosters comprehensive discussions about sexual health.
- Human immunodeficiency virus preexposure prophylaxis is safe and effective for LGBTQ + older adults.
- Substance use during sex is common and health-care providers play a critical role in mitigating risks.

INTRODUCTION

Sexuality, intimate activities, and the ability to express one's sexual identity contribute to a person's well-being and enjoyment in life.[1–3] An online survey of 6955 sexually diverse persons revealed that variances exist across sexual orientation groups in the context of casual sex but less so in long-term relationships. Gay cisgender men report the highest emotional and sexual satisfaction from casual sex while lesbian cisgender women were least satisfied by casual sex.[2] In a survey of 265 persons aged 60 to 75 years in same sex relationships, both cisgender men and women report high levels of sexual satisfaction that highly correlate with relationship satisfaction and resilience.[3] Most of these respondents were in long-term relationships and nearly three-quarters experienced complete monogamy. Other studies demonstrate greater variability of sexual satisfaction. A population-based study of 326 LGBTQ+ older adults compared to heterosexual counterparts revealed they were less likely to be married or cohabitating, report lower quality of life, and poorer life and sexual satisfaction even after correcting for socioeconomic factors.[4] Data

Department of Medicine, University of California San Diego, San Diego, CA, USA
* Corresponding author. 200 West Arbor Drive, Mail Code #8208, San Diego, CA 92103.
E-mail address: m1young@ucsd.edu

Clin Geriatr Med 40 (2024) 223–237
https://doi.org/10.1016/j.cger.2023.10.002
0749-0690/24/Published by Elsevier Inc.

from the National Social Life Health and Aging Project demonstrated that older gay and bisexual cisgender men (GBM) express more lack of interest in sex (48% vs 25%), report sex was not pleasurable (22% vs 6%), and experience anxiety around sexual performance (44% vs 26%) compared with heterosexual cisgender men.[5] Older cisgender women with same sex partners report less interest in sex than heterosexual cisgender women (15% vs 43%).

Multiple factors contribute to variability in sexual experiences by older Lesbian, Gay, Bisexual, Transgender, Queer and additional identities (LGBTQ +) adults including biologic health, psychological and emotional states, and anticipated and/or experienced negative life experiences.[6,7] Intersecting minority identifiers (eg, LGBTQ+, non-White race/ethnicity, and older age) may contribute to historical and ongoing experiences of trauma, perceived and enacted discrimination (including in the health-care sector), and ongoing invalidation.[8,9] The use of avoidant coping mechanisms such as substance use, disengagement in care, and condomless sex among others then affects an individual's physical, psychological, social, and sexual health (**Fig. 1**).[10] Overall, the sexual satisfaction and sexual health of older LGBTQ + individuals is shaped by experiences that occur throughout the life span. In this summary, we focus on current, pragmatic, and person-centered approaches to optimize the sexual health of the LGBTQ + older adults that we care for.

DISCUSSION

Optimizing the Sexual Health of LGBTQ + Older Adults

Despite the importance of sex to older adults, only 22% to 48% of cisgender men and 8% to 38% of cisgender women 50 years and older[5] report ever discussing sex with their

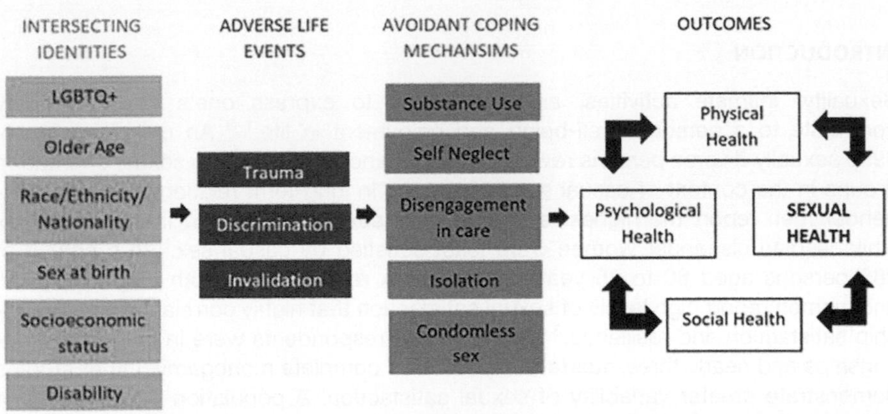

Fig. 1. Minority identities such as sexual/gender identity, age, race, sex at birth, socioeconomic status, or disability result in unique and negative stressors that occur during a life span. These often include traumatic experiences, discrimination, and invalidation/dehumanization. These adverse life experiences are magnified when minority identities intersect such as in LGBTQ + older adults (whom may have experienced a lifetime of negative experiences related to their gender and sexuality and are now facing the invalidating impact of ageism). To minimize the impact of ongoing adverse experiences, avoidance is frequently used that can manifest as substance use, neglect, disengagement, isolation, and unhealthy sexual behaviors. This contributes to poorer psychological, physical, and social health, all of which in turn influence sexual health. The implementation of culturally competent, person-centered care is validating leading to LGBTQ + older adult empowerment to strive for improved psychological, physical, social, and sexual health.

health-care provider.[5,11] In fact, 20% of LGBTQ+ adults 50 years and older are not "out" to their primary physician.[12,13] Common barriers to care include recent experiences of stigma and discrimination, fear that disclosure may contribute to adverse health outcomes, lack of perceived LGBTQ + cultural competence among health-care providers, and limited health literacy of LGBTQ + persons.[14,15]

Small changes to the built environment can go a long way toward welcoming diverse persons. Examples include visual cues in the clinical environment (eg, diverse representation on flyers and magazines), inclusive restroom access[16]; and implementation of chosen name and pronouns in clinical encounters and medical records.[17] However, what matters most is the interpersonal interactions that contribute to an environment of respect, foster trust, and empower LGBTQ + persons.[18,19] We recommend implementing approaches including introducing yourself with pronouns; soliciting lived names and gender pronouns; asking respectful, nonjudgmental questions; and devoting time to listening, learning, and validating their personhood.[18,19] When discussing sexual health concerns consider using the 10 P's of taking a sexual history (**Table 1**).[20] This starts by discussing the reason for the line of questioning and asking *permission* to have the conversation, an approach that empowers the individual to proceed or not. Some questions will elicit *preferences* regarding how they view/label their anatomic organs (penis, testes, prostate, chest/breasts, vagina, cervix, uterus,

Table 1
Culturally competent sexual history using the 10 Ps

10 Ps	Example Questions
Preface/permission	Sexual health impacts quality of life, would you be willing to talk to me about that?
Preferences	Do you have any language that you prefer to use when talking about your genitals (eg, your vagina vs the vagina vs the front hole)? Also enables documentation of anatomic/organ inventory at any given time.[a]
Partners	What are the gender identities of your partners? Do you know if your partners are only having sex with you? Do you ever pay or trade for sex?
Practices	What types of sex (eg, vaginal, anal, oral, toys, groups, other) do you engage in?
Pharmaceuticals	Do you use any drugs either prescribed or not prescribed during sex? [b]
Protection from STIs	Are there some types of sex where you do not use condoms or other barriers? What are your reasons for that?
Past history of STIs	Have you ever had an STI? If so, do you remember the site (eg, throat, vagina, and anus)?
Pregnancy	Are you or your partner interested in having children? [c]
Pleasure	Do you have concerns about being able to become and sustain arousal during sex? Is sex painful or uncomfortable?
Partner violence	Has anyone ever forced you to do anything sexually that you did not want to do?

[a] Persons may prefer gender-neutral terms (eg, chest instead of breast).
[b] This is also an opportunity to explore injection drug use in persons not having sex, a risk factor for HIV and hepatitis B/C acquisition.
[c] Older adults may have much younger partners and thus may be interested in starting a family.
Adapted from Prevention CfDCa. A Guide to Taking a Sexual History. Updated January 14, 2022. Accessed August 30, 2023, 2023.

and ovaries); the gender identities of *partners*; the types of sexual *practices* they engage in and whether or not they use *pharmaceuticals* (illicit or prescribed) during sex. We then follow up with exploring *protection* from and *past history* of sexually transmitted infections (STIs) to understand the need for additional laboratory testing and provide recommendations to optimize sexual health. We still explore *pregnancy* because partners may be younger and have desires and questions around starting a family. Finally, we inquire about *pleasure* and *partner violence* because these are often sensitive to discuss and may require more time commitment. Sexual pleasure is dependent on multiple factors including psychological (eg, mental health),[21,22] physical (eg, co-occurring conditions, medications, normal age-related changes, whether they are status post gender-affirming surgery),[23–26] and social (eg, self-perception, internalized stigma)[27] health. Exploring the impact of these different domains enables health-care providers to identify modifiable factors including treatment of depression, provision of medications/hormone replacement therapy for erectile dysfunction or vaginal dryness, and validation in the context of internalized stigma (related to age, LGBTQ+, race, and so forth). The LGBTQ + community are highly heterogeneous, thus rates of intimate partner violence (IPV) are variable but do seem to be higher than for heterosexual persons.[28] Reports suggest that GBM demonstrate a 5-year rate of 22% of physical abuse and 5.1% of sexual abuse, which is similar to a survey of mixed-sex cohabitating cisgender women (5-year rate of 20.4% physical abuse and 4.4% sexual abuse).[29] Other LGBTQ + communities experience even higher rates as transgender individuals have a lifetime physical IPV rate of 37.5% and sexual IPV of 25%.[30] Unique expressions of IPV include partners threatening "outing" an individual, whereas internalized gender minority stigma may lead LGBTQ + persons to remain in abusive relationships.[31] Nearly no data exists that characterize the risk of IPV for LGBTQ + older adults but studies do document significant and negative consequences including chronic pain, anxiety/depression, increased risk of human immunodeficiency virus (HIV), and a 300% higher mortality rate.[32,33] Overall, LGBTQ+ and heterosexual older adults have similar sexual health needs and the delivery of culturally competent care is key.[11]

Preventing Sexually Transmitted Infections in LGBTQ + Older Adults

The epidemiology of human immunodeficiency virus in older adults

Current US Preventive Services Task Force recommendations include routine HIV testing for persons aged 15 to 65 years.[34] This recommendation is provided with the caveat that adults aged older than 65 years who are at an increased risk of HIV infection should be screened with screening intervals (eg, twice a year, once a year) depending on individual reported risks.[35] In 2019, 10% of all new HIV diagnoses occurred in persons aged 55 years and older, representing 9% of all new diagnoses in cisgender men but 17% of all new diagnoses in cisgender women. More recent advancements such as potent, convenient, and well-tolerated antiretroviral therapy and HIV preexposure prophylaxis (PrEP) are decreasing new HIV infections across most age groups except for ages 25 to 34 and 55 years and older. Most importantly, persons aged 55 years and older are often diagnosed later into their HIV infection resulting in higher risk of acquired immunodeficiency syndrome at diagnosis.[36]

Several surveys demonstrate that as age increases, condom use decreases.[37,38] Among sexually active persons aged 50 years and older, 37% of GBM report inconsistent condom use compared to 27%[39] of heterosexual cisgender men and 35% of heterosexual cisgender women.[40] Many reasons exist for decreasing use of condoms with age including higher prioritization of sexual pleasure (in the context of erectile dysfunction and vaginal dryness) and companionship over concern for STIs.[41–43]

The variability of condomless sex in studies highlights the importance of talking to older adults of all sexual orientations about their sexual health to provide education and recommendations that ensure sex is enjoyable and safer. LGBTQ + older adults may also not perceive themselves at risk for STIs, even in the context of new sex partners related to relationship changes that may accompany the transition to later life.[37,44] PrEP for HIV prevention should be discussed especially when condom or other barrier use is inconsistent.

Human immunodeficiency virus preexposure prophylaxis in older adults

PrEP is a safe and empowering strategy that prevents HIV in heterosexual individuals, GBM, transgender women (TGW), and people who inject drugs.[45–47] To date 3 options are available: (1) oral tenofovir disoproxil fumarate with emtricitabine (TDF/FTC), (2) oral tenofovir alafenamide with emtricitabine (TAF/emtrictiabine [FTC]) for cisgender men and TGW engaging in anal sex,[48,49] and (3) injectable cabotegravir (CAB) every 2 months.[50,51] Even though few older adults were included in the clinical trials establishing the safety and efficacy of PrEP, this should not dissuade health-care providers from its use. The US Preventive Services Task Force (USPSTF) advises that all individuals at high risk for HIV infection be provided PrEP (Grade A).[52] Detailed guidelines exist for the provision of PrEP so we will focus on common questions and clinical pearls.[53]

When to recommend preexposure prophylaxis in LGBTQ + older adult human immunodeficiency virus serodiscordant couples

PrEP is not medically indicated in LGBTQ + older adults in exclusive nonpolyamorous relationships where the partner living with HIV is taking their antiretroviral therapy consistently and maintains an undetectable HIV viral load. Extensive evidence exists that when persons living with HIV maintain an undetectable HIV viral load (defined as < 200 copies/mL), they will not transmit HIV.[54] However, in serodiscordant couples, the additional use of PrEP may enhance coping with HIV serodiscordance and decrease anxiety when engaging in sex.[55,56] Our practice is to use a person-centered approach in discussions with serodiscordant couples with the goal of optimizing sexual intimacy for both persons while monitoring potential health risks to the person on PrEP.

What do I need to consider when starting or stopping preexposure prophylaxis?

Laboratory screening for PrEP primarily involves ensuring that the person is not already living with HIV. This is done by documenting a Food and Drug Administration (FDA)-approved negative HIV antigen/antibody blood or point of care test 1 week prior to initiation *and* confirming no signs or symptoms of a recent viral infection (eg, fever, fatigue, myalgias, rash, headache, pharyngitis, lymphadenopathy, arthralgias, night sweats, or diarrhea) if condomless sex and/or injection drug use occurred within the last 30 days. If symptoms are present, consider deferring PrEP, ordering a plasma HIV-1 RNA assay, and repeating in 2 to 4 weeks if negative. If the HIV exposure event is within the past 72 hours and HIV risk is ongoing, consider initiating HIV nonoccupational postexposure prophylaxis (PEP). The first visit also includes evaluating for other STIs (syphilis, gonorrhea, chlamydia, and hepatitis C virus), testing for immunity to hepatitis B virus (HBV), and evaluating renal function and lipids. Along with the prevention of HIV infection, TDF and TAF are also active against HBV, and abrupt discontinuation in the context of chronic active HBV may result in HBV DNA reactivation and hepatitis flares.[57] Worldwide, LGBTQ+ persons demonstrate an overall higher prevalence of HBV infection compared to the general population and may be at higher risk for this uncommon but serious complication.[58] Medications used for PrEP are well tolerated; however, TDF can infrequently cause acute tubular toxicity (Fanconi syndrome) resulting in renal failure, vitamin D deficiency, hypophosphatemia, osteomalacia, bone pain, and fractures.[59,60] In the context of TDF use for PrEP, initial drops in estimated glomerular filtration rates do occur but progressive renal impairment is uncommon.[60,61] TAF is a prodrug resulting in lower circulating plasma levels of tenofovir translating to much lower rates of renal toxicity.[62] However, there are higher rates of weight gain and elevated low-density lipid levels compared to TDF.[63] Due to these differences TDF/FTC should not be used in persons with estimated creatinine clearances (eCrCl) less than 60 mL/min and TAF/FTC in persons with eCrCl less than 30 mL/min. Current guidelines do not recommend monitoring for osteopenia but one retrospective study suggests TDF/FTC is associated with a higher risk of developing osteopenia/osteoporosis, and we recommend pursuing bone mineral density testing if additional contributors (eg, postmenopausal state, underweight, and frailty phenotype) are present.[64]

A third option is long-acting CAB. CAB initiation includes gluteal muscle injections every 2 months with an optional daily oral lead-in 30 days prior to injections. Because of the long duration of drug exposure with CAB, a HIV-1 RNA assay should be performed within 1 week of initiation to rule out very recent HIV infection. Discontinuation of CAB results in a prolonged period of waning drug levels (referred to as the “tail period”) placing individuals at risk of developing drug-resistant HIV if acquired. Thus, discontinuing CAB in persons with ongoing HIV exposures requires starting a reliable highly effective HIV prevention method.

Another potential approach to minimize kidney and bone toxicities of PrEP, in older cisgender men who have sex with men (MSM) reporting rare condomless sexual encounters is “2-1-1” or “on-demand” PrEP.[65,66] Although not an FDA-approved regimen, studies demonstrate that 2 tablets of TDF/FTC 2 to 24 hours before sex plus 1 pill 24 hours after the initial 2 pill dose and 1 pill 48 hours after the initial 2 pill dose is effective in reducing HIV acquisition in MSM. It is important to note that “2-1-1” has only been evaluated with TDF/FTC and cannot translate to TAF/FTC. Additionally, this regimen should not be used in persons with concurrent chronic HBV.

Prevention of other sexually transmitted infections for LGBTQ + older adults

Bacterial STIs (eg, *Neisseria gonorrhoeae*, *Chlamydia trachomatis*, and *Treponema pallidum*) have steadily increased in GBM.[67] Doxycycline as PrEP or PEP has been studied because it is an antibiotic that has a moderate spectrum of coverage, is well tolerated, and is rapidly absorbed via the oral route and is a generic drug.[68] Several randomized clinical trials using doxycycline for STI postexposure prophylaxis (Doxy PEP) demonstrate significantly decreased incidences of chlamydia, syphilis, and to a lesser degree gonorrhea (effect depends on regional doxycycline resistance) in MSM and TGW.[65,69] Despite the apparent benefits of Doxy PEP, limited information is known about long-term effects including individual health risks (eg, changes to the microbiome) and community level antimicrobial resistance.[70,71] To date, there are no official endorsements from the USA International Antiviral Society, Centers for Disease Control and Prevention, or the World Health Organization.[72] The British Organization for Sexual Health and HIV and the UK Health Security Agency do not endorse use of doxycycline for PEP or PrEP.[73] Other limitations of current studies include minimal to no participation of GBM and TGW aged 50 years and older. Concern also exists that older GBM and TGW may be at greater risk for doxycycline-associated adverse effects such as photosensitivity, benign intracranial hypertension, and gastrointestinal distress including esophagitis.[74] Despite an overall lukewarm reception from national health organizations, we include Doxy PEP in our discussion because it is being used

Table 2
Drugs commonly associated with chemsex

	Street or Brand Names	Common routes	Pharmacologic properties	Characteristics
Most commonly reported or classic chemsex drugs				
Methamphetamine	Christina, crystal, crystal meth, ice, meth, and Tina	Smoked, snorted, injected (intravenously or anally) or inserted into urethra	Stimulant	Amphetamine-type stimulants; became more common in the 1990s as an ingredient in MDMA pills to improve endurance, can facilitate disinhibition, increase arousal, and sexual adventurism
GHB and GBL	G, Gina, G water, and liquid ecstasy	Swallowed	Depressant	Emerged in the early 1990s; can induce euphoria; acute intoxication is a key risk due to a narrow safety window
Mephedrone	Bath salts, drone, Mcat, meow meow, and 4–MMC	Smoked, snorted, injected (intravenously or intramuscularly), or swallowed	Stimulant	Firs synthesized in 1920s; can induce euphoria, elevated mood, and increased sexual performance; currently used mostly in the English-speaking countries but becoming more common as an alternative to methamphetamine due to its lower price and less legal restrictions for some synthetic cathinone
Other drugs also considered part of the chemsex scene in some regions				
Ketamine	K, special K, and vitamin K	Smoked or snorted	Depressant, dissociative	Used as an anesthetic agent originally; induces a dissociative state with visual and auditory hallucinations
MDMA	E, ecstasy, Mandy, Molly, and XTC	Swallowed	Stimulant	Widely used as a recreational drug since 1980s; induces feelings of euphoria, energy, happiness, and desire to socialize

(*continued on next page*)

Table 2
(*continued*)

	Street or Brand Names	Common routes	Pharmacologic properties	Characteristics
Cocaine	Coca, coke, crack, snow, and stash	Smoked or snorted	Stimulant	Facilitates enhanced feelings of energy, confidence, exhilaration, and sociability
Substances commonly used alongside but not typically constituting chemsex drugs				
Alkyl nitrates	Bolt, poppers, and rush	Snorted	Vasodilator	Relaxes vascular smooth muscles; used in sexual settings since the 1970s in various populations such as adolescents, MSM, and people who visit nightclubs
Cannabis or marijuana	420, grass, has, herb, pot, and weed	Smoked or swallowed	Cannabimimetic	Used for both medicinal and recreational purposes; desired effect includes euphoria, sedation, relaxation, and increased sexual arousal
Sildenafil, tadalafil, and vardenafil	Viagra, Cialis, and Levitra	Swallowed	Vasodilator	Brand and generic drugs for treating erectile dysfunction; used in chemsex to offset erection problems associated with high-dose methamphetamine and oral PrEP (emtricitabine and TDF)

Abbreviations: GBL, γ-butyrolactone; GHB, γ-hydroxybutyrate; MDMA, 3,4-methylenedioxymethamphetamine; 4-MMC, 4-methylmethcathinone.

off-label for MSM and TGW and includes individuals who purchase and use doxycycline without a prescription.[70,71]

Addressing Chemsex in LGBTQ + Older Adults

LGBTQ + older adults may experience complicated relationships with substance use (including tobacco, marijuana, and alcohol).[72,75] Sexualized drug use (SDU) also known as "Chemsex" is defined as the use of any illicit drug prior to and during sex for the purpose of initiating, prolonging, and intensifying the experience.[76] Chemsex predominantly affects MSM with a prevalence ranging from 3% to 29%, depending on context and sampling.[77] Methamphetamine, mephedrone, and gamma hydroxybutyrate/gamma-butyrolactone (GHB/GBL) are most commonly associated with chemsex with cocaine, ketamine, and 3,4-methlenedioxymeth-amphetamine (MDMA) being less common.[78] Characteristics of commonly used drugs are further detailed in **Table 2**.[79] Chemsex is often paired with erectile dysfunction drugs and is associated with increased condomless anal sex.[80,81] MSM disclosing chemsex were more likely to have a recent bacterial STI, rectal STI, or hepatitis C compared to those not participating in chemsex.[82] Chemsex was also associated with more sexual partners, transactional sex, group sex, sharing sex toys, injection drug use, higher alcohol consumption, and subsequent use of PEP for HIV. Demographic data from studies suggest that older MSM are participating in chemsex but perhaps at lower rates than younger MSM (27%–33% of persons aged 45 years and older attending a sexual health clinic).[83] Narratives investigating the use of chemsex in older MSM suggest it is used to enhance sociality in the context of loneliness.[84,85] We recommend not only inquiring about chemsex with LGBTQ + older adults but also inquiring the reasoning behind its use to codevelop and implement harm reduction interventions (eg, sterile intravenous needles, naloxone, and medication-assisted treatment) and alternate coping approaches (eg, joining group exercise, social clubs, and so forth).

SUMMARY

In summary, sexual health is important to LGBTQ + older adults. As health-care providers, we can use culturally competent care and create inclusive and welcoming clinic environments that enable education and empowerment of LGBTQ + older adults so they can pursue their sexual interests in healthy and safe ways. This may include HIV PrEP, other STIs preventive approaches and strategies to mitigate the risks of SDU.

CLINICS CARE POINTS

- The LGBTQ + older adult community is diverse, and discussions around sex and sexual health should avoid assumptions and be person centered.
- HIV PrEP is a highly effective preventative intervention that should be used in older adults that report HIV risk factors (condomless sex unless with monogamous partner and injection drug use).
  - TDF/FTC is a daily oral pill that can be used in *all persons*.
  - TAF/FTC is a daily oral pill only approved for *cisgender men and transwomen participating in anal sex*.
  - CAB is an injectable PrEP that is provided every 2 months for *all persons*. CAB is a long-acting medication, and discontinuation requires starting a reliable highly active HIV-prevention approach (usually TDF/FTC or TAF/FTC).

- Studies demonstrate the benefit of doxycycline 200 mg po within 72 hours (ideally within 24 hours) after condomless sex to decrease the risk of acquiring chlamydia, syphilis, and gonorrhea (eg, Doxy PEP). Global health organizations have not yet endorsed Doxy PEP due to unknowns around the long-term impact of this strategy on individuals' microbiomes, antimicrobial resistance, and the frequency of other side effects.
- SDU or chemsex is common among MSM. Providers should inquire and work with older LGBTQ + adults who participate in chemsex to mitigate risks of STIs acquisition and other negative health effects of substance use.

DISCLOSURE

M.Y. Karris has received past funding to the institution for independent research projects from Gilead Sciences and ViiV Healthcare.

FUNDING

This publication resulted in part from research supported by the San Diego Center for AIDS Research (SD CFAR), an NIH-funded program (P30 AI036214), which is supported by the following NIH Institutes and Centers: NIAID, NCI, NHLBI, NIA, NICHD, NIDA, NIDCR, NIDDK, NIMH, NIMHD, NINR, FIC, and OAR.

REFERENCES

1. Smith L, Yang L, Veronese N, et al. Sexual activity is associated with greater enjoyment of life in older adults. Sex Med 2019;7(1):11–8.
2. Mark KP, Garcia JR, Fisher HE. Perceived emotional and sexual satisfaction across sexual relationship contexts: gender and sexual orientation differences and similarities. Can J Hum Sex 2015;24(2):120–30.
3. Fleishman JM, Crane B, Koch PB. Correlates and predictors of sexual satisfaction for older adults in same-sex relationships. J Homosex 2020;67(14):1974–98.
4. Grabovac I, Smith L, McDermott DT, et al. Well-being among older gay and bisexual men and women in England: a cross-sectional population study. J Am Med Dir Assoc 2019;20(9):1080–5, e1.
5. Brennan-Ing M, Kaufman JE, Larson B, et al. Sexual health among lesbian, gay, bisexual, and heterosexual older adults: an exploratory analysis. Clin Gerontol 2021;44(3):222–34.
6. Hoy-Ellis CP, Fredriksen-Goldsen KI. Lesbian, gay, & bisexual older adults: linking internal minority stressors, chronic health conditions, and depression. Aging Ment Health 2016;20(11):1119–30.
7. Meyer IH. Prejudice, social stress, and mental health in lesbian, gay, and bisexual populations: conceptual issues and research evidence. Psychol Bull 2003; 129(5):674.
8. Scheer JR, Antebi-Gruszka N. A psychosocial risk model of potentially traumatic events and sexual risk behavior among LGBTQ individuals. J Trauma & Dissociation 2019;20(5):603–18.
9. Mandelbaum J. Advancing health equity by integrating intersectionality into epidemiological research: applications and challenges. J Epidemiol Community Health 2020;74(9):761–2.
10. Gessner M, Bishop MD, Martos A, et al. Sexual minority people's perspectives of sexual health care: understanding minority stress in sexual health settings. Sex Res Soc Pol 2020;17:607–18.

11. Lindau ST, Schumm LP, Laumann EO, et al. A study of sexuality and health among older adults in the United States. N Engl J Med 2007;357(8):762–74.
12. Fredriksen-Goldsen KI, Kim H-J, Emlet CA, et al. The aging and health report. Seattle, WA: Institute for Multigenerational Health; 2011.
13. Hughes M. Health and well being of lesbian, gay, bisexual, transgender and intersex people aged 50 years and over. Aust Health Rev 2017;42(2):146 51.
14. Alba B, Lyons A, Waling A, et al. Older lesbian and gay adults' perceptions of barriers and facilitators to accessing health and aged care services in Australia. Health Soc Care Community 2021;29(4):918–27.
15. Portz JD, Retrum JH, Wright LA, et al. Assessing capacity for providing culturally competent services to LGBT older adults. In: Lesbian, Gay, Bisexual, and Transgender Aging, Routledge, UK, 2017, 231–247.
16. Herman JL. Gendered restrooms and minority stress: the public regulation of gender and its impact on transgender people's lives. J Publ Manag Soc Pol 2013;19(1):65.
17. Davison K, Queen R, Lau F, et al. Culturally competent gender, sex, and sexual orientation information practices and electronic health records: rapid review. JMIR Medical Informatics 2021;9(2):e25467.
18. Hudson KD, Bruce-Miller V. Nonclinical best practices for creating LGBTQ-inclusive care environments: a scoping review of gray literature. J Gay Lesb Soc Serv 2023;35(2):218–40.
19. McClain Z, Hawkins LA, Yehia BR. Creating welcoming spaces for lesbian, gay, bisexual, and transgender (LGBT) patients: an evaluation of the health care environment. J Homosex 2016;63(3):387–93.
20. Prevention CfDCa. A Guide to Taking a Sexual History. Updated January 14, 2022. https://www.cdc.gov/std/treatment/sexualhistory.htm. Accessed August 30, 2023, 2023.
21. Laurent SM, Simons AD. Sexual dysfunction in depression and anxiety: conceptualizing sexual dysfunction as part of an internalizing dimension. Clin Psychol Rev 2009;29(7):573–85.
22. Michael A, O'Keane V. Sexual dysfunction in depression. Hum Psychopharmacol Clin Exp 2000;15(5):337–45.
23. Bener A, Al-Hamaq AO, Kamran S, et al. Prevalence of erectile dysfunction in male stroke patients, and associated co-morbidities and risk factors. Int Urol Nephrol 2008;40:701–8.
24. Rosen RC. Prevalence and risk factors of sexual dysfunction in men and women. Curr Psychiatr Rep 2000;2(3):189–95.
25. Hayes R, Dennerstein L. The impact of aging on sexual function and sexual dysfunction in women: a review of population-based studies. J Sex Med 2005; 2(3):317–30.
26. Schardein JN, Nikolavsky D. Sexual functioning of transgender females post-vaginoplasty: evaluation, outcomes and treatment strategies for sexual dysfunction. Sexual Medicine Reviews 2022;10(1):77–90.
27. Budge SL, Katz-Wise SL. Sexual minorities' gender norm conformity and sexual satisfaction: the mediating effects of sexual communication, internalized stigma, and sexual narcissism. Int J Sex Health 2019;31(1):36–49.
28. Ard KL, Makadon HJ. Addressing intimate partner violence in lesbian, gay, bisexual, and transgender patients. J Gen Intern Med 2011;26:930–3.
29. Tjaden PG, Extent. nature, and consequences of intimate partner violence. USA: US Department of Justice, Office of Justice Programs, National Institute; 2000.

30. Peitzmeier SM, Malik M, Kattari SK, et al. Intimate partner violence in transgender populations: systematic review and meta-analysis of prevalence and correlates. American Journal of Public Health 2020;110(9):e1–14.
31. Kulkin HS, Williams J, Borne HF, et al. A review of research on violence in same-gender couples: a resource for clinicians. J Homosex 2007;53(4):71–87.
32. Hillman J. Intimate partner violence among older LGBT adults: unique risk factors, issues in reporting and treatment, and recommendations for research, practice, and policy. Intimate partner violence and the LGBT+ community: understanding power. dynamics 2020;237–54.
33. Dong X, Simon M, De Leon CM, et al. Elder self-neglect and abuse and mortality risk in a community-dwelling population. JAMA 2009;302(5):517–26.
34. 2023 Final Recommendation Statement Human Immunodeficiency Virus (HIV) Infection: Screening (2019).
35. 2023 HIV by Age (2020). Available at: https://www.cdc.gov/hiv/pdf/library/reports/surveillance/cdc-hiv-surveillance-supplemental-report-vol-26-1.pdf.
36. Mugavero MJ, Castellano C, Edelman D, et al. Late diagnosis of HIV infection: the role of age and sex. Am J Med 2007;120(4):370–3.
37. Fisher L. Sex, romance, and relationships: AARP survey of midlife and older adults. AARP. 2010 2016.
38. Reece M, Herbenick D, Schick V, et al. Condom use rates in a national probability sample of males and females ages 14 to 94 in the United States. J Sex Med 2010; 7:266–76.
39. Fonner VA, Dalglish SL, Kennedy CE, et al. Effectiveness and safety of oral HIV preexposure prophylaxis for all populations. AIDS (London, England) 2016; 30(12):1973.
40. Lovejoy TI, Heckman TG, Sikkema KJ, et al. Patterns and correlates of sexual activity and condom use behavior in persons 50-plus years of age living with HIV/AIDS. AIDS Behav 2008;12:943–56.
41. DeLamater J, Koepsel E. In: Relationships and sexual expression in later life: a biopsychosocial perspective, Sexuality & Ageing. 1st edition. UK: Routledge; 2017. p. 49–71.
42. Taylor TN, Munoz-Plaza CE, Goparaju L, et al. “The pleasure is better as I’ve gotten older”: sexual health, sexuality, and sexual risk behaviors among older women living with HIV. Arch Sex Behav 2017;46:1137–50.
43. Gewirtz-Meydan A, Ayalon L. Why do older adults have sex? Approach and avoidance sexual motives among older women and men. J Sex Res 2019;56(7):870–81.
44. Syme ML, Cohn TJ, Barnack-Tavlaris J. A comparison of actual and perceived sexual risk among older adults. J Sex Res 2017;54(2):149–60.
45. Grant RM, Lama JR, Anderson PL, et al. Preexposure chemoprophylaxis for HIV prevention in men who have sex with men. N Engl J Med 2010;363(27):2587–99.
46. Thigpen MC, Kebaabetswe PM, Paxton LA, et al. Antiretroviral preexposure prophylaxis for heterosexual HIV transmission in. N Engl J Med 2012;367(5):423–34.
47. Baeten JM, Donnell D, Ndase P, et al. Antiretroviral prophylaxis for HIV prevention in heterosexual men and women. N Engl J Med 2012;367(5):399–410.
48. Mayer KH, Molina J-M, Thompson MA, et al. Emtricitabine and tenofovir alafenamide vs emtricitabine and tenofovir disoproxil fumarate for HIV pre-exposure prophylaxis (DISCOVER): primary results from a randomised, double-blind, multicentre, active-controlled, phase 3, non-inferiority trial. Lancet 2020;396(10246):239–54.
49. Ruane P, Clarke A, Post FA, et al. Phase 3 randomized, controlled DISCOVER study of daily F/TAF or F/TDF for HIV pre-exposure prophylaxis: week 96 results.

InProgram and abstracts of the 17th European AIDS Conference, Basel, Switserland 2019 Nov 6. (Conference abstract)
50. Landovitz RJ, Donnell D, Clement ME, et al. Cabotegravir for HIV prevention in cisgender men and transgender women. N Engl J Med 2021;385(7):595–608.
51. Mitchell KM, Boily M-C, Hanscom B, et al. Estimating the impact of HIV PrEP regimens containing long-acting injectable cabotegravir or daily oral tenofovir disoproxil fumarate/emtricitabine among men who have sex with men in the United States: a mathematical modelling study for HPTN 083. Lancet Regional Health–Americas 2023;4:100416.
52. Walensky RP, Paltiel AD. New USPSTF Guidelines for HIV screening and preexposure prophylaxis (PrEP): straight A's. JAMA Netw Open 2019;2(6):e195042.
53. UPST Force, Owens DK, Davidson KW, et al. Pre exposure prophylaxis for the prevention of HIV infection: US preventive services task force recommendation statement. JAMA, J Am Med Assoc 2019;321(22):2203–13.
54. Eisinger RW, Dieffenbach CW, Fauci AS. HIV viral load and transmissibility of HIV infection: undetectable equals untransmittable. JAMA 2019;321(5):451–2.
55. Ngure K, Heffron R, Curran K, et al. I knew I would be safer. Experiences of Kenyan HIV serodiscordant couples soon after pre-exposure prophylaxis (PrEP) initiation. AIDS Patient Care and STDs 2016;30(2):78–83.
56. Brooks RA, Landovitz RJ, Kaplan RL, et al. Sexual risk behaviors and acceptability of HIV pre-exposure prophylaxis among HIV-negative gay and bisexual men in serodiscordant relationships: a mixed methods study. AIDS patient care and STDs 2012;26(2):87–94.
57. Mohareb AM, Larmarange J, Kim AY, et al. Risks and benefits of oral HIV pre-exposure prophylaxis for people with chronic hepatitis B. Lancet HIV 2022;9(8):e585–94.
58. Moradi G, Soheili M, Rashti R, et al. The prevalence of hepatitis C and hepatitis B in lesbian, gay, bisexual and transgender populations: a systematic review and meta-analysis. European Journal of Medical Research 2022;27(1):47.
59. Tourret J, Deray G, Isnard-Bagnis C. Tenofovir effect on the kidneys of HIV-infected patients: a double-edged sword? J Am Soc Nephrol: JASN (J Am Soc Nephrol) 2013;24(10):1519.
60. Pilkington V, Hill A, Hughes S, et al. How safe is TDF/FTC as PrEP? A systematic review and meta-analysis of the risk of adverse events in 13 randomised trials of PrEP. Journal of Virus Eradication 2018;4(4):215–24.
61. Mugwanya KK, Wyatt C, Celum C, et al. Reversibility of glomerular renal function decline in HIV uninfected men and women discontinuing emtricitabine-tenofovir disoproxil fumarate pre-exposure prophylaxis. J Acquir Immune Defic Syndr (1999) 2016;71(4):374.
62. DeJesus E, Haas B, Segal-Maurer S, et al. Superior efficacy and improved renal and bone safety after switching from a tenofovir disoproxil fumarate-to a tenofovir alafenamide-based regimen through 96 weeks of treatment. AIDS Res Hum Retrovir 2018;34(4):337–42.
63. Kauppinen KJ, Aho I, Sutinen J. Switching from tenofovir alafenamide to tenofovir disoproxil fumarate improves lipid profile and protects from weight gain. AIDS 2022;36(10):1337–44.
64. Chang J, Do D, Delgado H, et al. A retrospective analysis of bone loss in tenofovir-emtricitabine therapy for HIV PrEP. Int J STD AIDS 2022;33(14):1183–92.
65. Molina JM, Capitant C, Spire B, et al. On-Demand Preexposure Prophylaxis in Men at High Risk for HIV-1 Infection. N Engl J Med 2015;373(23):2237–46.

66. Antoni G, Tremblay C, Delaugerre C, et al. On-demand pre-exposure prophylaxis with tenofovir disoproxil fumarate plus emtricitabine among men who have sex with men with less frequent sexual intercourse: a post-hoc analysis of the ANRS IPERGAY trial. Lancet HIV 2020;7(2):e113–20.
67. Bowen VB, Braxton J, Davis DW, et al. Sexually transmitted disease surveillance 2018. (goverment document). 2019.
68. Grant JS, Stafylis C, Celum C, et al. Doxycycline prophylaxis for bacterial sexually transmitted infections. Clin Infect Dis 2020;70(6):1247–53.
69. Luetkemeyer AF, Donnell D, Dombrowski JC, et al. Postexposure doxycycline to prevent bacterial sexually transmitted infections. N Engl J Med 2023;388(14): 1296–306.
70. Unemo M, Kong FYS. Doxycycline-PEP—novel and promising but needs monitoring. Nat Rev Urol 2023;1–2.
71. Kong FYS, Kenyon C, Unemo M. Important considerations regarding the widespread use of doxycycline chemoprophylaxis against sexually transmitted infections. J Antimicrob Chemother 2023;78:dkad129.
72. Pantoja-Patiño JR. The socio-multidimensional sexual and gender minority oppression framework: a model for LGBTQ individuals experiencing oppression and substance use. J LGBT Issues Couns 2020;14(3):268–83.
73. Kohli M, Medland N, Fifer H, et al. BASHH updated position statement on doxycycline as prophylaxis for sexually transmitted infections. Chicago, USA: BMJ Publishing Group Ltd; 2022.
74. Eljaaly K, Alghamdi H, Almehmadi H, et al. Long-term gastrointestinal adverse effects of doxycycline. Journal of Infection in Developing Countries 2023;17(02): 281–5.
75. Stall R, Purcell DW. Intertwining epidemics: a review of research on substance use among men who have sex with men and its connection to the AIDS epidemic. AIDS Behav 2000;4:181–92.
76. Bourne A, Reid D, Hickson F, et al. Illicit drug use in sexual settings ('chemsex') and HIV/STI transmission risk behaviour among gay men in South London: findings from a qualitative study. Sex Transm Infect 2015;91(8):564–8.
77. Maxwell S, Shahmanesh M, Gafos M. Chemsex behaviours among men who have sex with men: a systematic review of the literature. Int J Drug Pol 2019; 63:74–89.
78. Frankis J, Flowers P, McDaid L, et al. Low levels of chemsex among men who have sex with men, but high levels of risk among men who engage in chemsex: analysis of a cross-sectional online survey across four countries. Sex Health 2018;15(2):144–50.
79. Strong C, Huang P, Li C-W, et al. HIV, chemsex, and the need for harm-reduction interventions to support gay, bisexual, and other men who have sex with men. Lancet HIV 2022;9:E717–25.
80. Hibbert MP, Brett CE, Porcellato LA, et al. Psychosocial and sexual characteristics associated with sexualised drug use and chemsex among men who have sex with men (MSM) in the UK. Sex Transm Infect 2019;95(5):342–50.
81. Pufall E, Kall M, Shahmanesh M, et al. Sexualized drug use ('chemsex') and high-risk sexual behaviours in HIV-positive men who have sex with men. HIV Med 2018;19(4):261–70.
82. Hegazi A, Lee M, Whittaker W, et al. Chemsex and the city: sexualised substance use in gay bisexual and other men who have sex with men attending sexual health clinics. Int J STD AIDS 2017;28(4):362–6.

83. Drückler S, van Rooijen MS, de Vries HJ. Chemsex among men who have sex with men: a sexualized drug use survey among clients of the sexually transmitted infection outpatient clinic and users of a gay dating app in Amsterdam, The Netherlands. Sex Transm Dis 2018;45(5):325.
84. Di Feliciantonio C. Chemsex among gay men living with HIV aged over 45 in England and Italy: sociality and pleasure in times of undetectability. HIV, sex and sexuality in later life. Policy Press; 2022. p. 67–83.
85. McCullagh C, I'm not fragile like the new-age kids," Aging positively and reducing risk among older adults with HIV/AIDS: a qualitative and quantitative exploration. Columbia University; Bristol, UK.

Medical Issues Affecting Older Gay and Bisexual Men

Michael Danielewicz, MD

KEYWORDS

• Equity • Inclusion • Older • Gay • Bisexual • LGBTQIA+ • MSM

KEY POINTS

- Older gay and bisexual men have lived through defining historical moments of the twentieth century, including the human immunodeficiency virus (HIV) epidemic.
- Older gay men report worse physical health compared with heterosexual counterparts; they have higher rates of alcohol and tobacco use and continue to be disproportionately affected by HIV.
- Physicians should be mindful of unique needs of older gay and bisexual adults in terms of mental health and cancer screenings.

INTRODUCTION

LGBTQ+ older adults represent sizable, diverse, and potentially vulnerable populations; even the definition of what constitutes "older" varies, generally ranging from ages 50 to 65+ years depending on the source. Gay and bisexual men are two such groups that have historically faced inequities, both socially and medically; they have also demonstrated the resilience shown by lesbian, gay, bisexual, transgender, queer, and expansive identities (LGBTQ)+ communities across modern American history.

Gay and bisexual older men came of age in eras defined by heteronormativity and have witnessed shifting societal views on sexuality and gender identity. As they aged, many saw, participated in, and were affected by major societal phenomena of the twentieth century. From the 1940s to the 1960s, their ability to participate in government roles was threatened as the "Lavender Scare" sought out and fired gay and bisexual government workers; these "sexual sociopaths" were seen not just as mentally ill, but also as a threat to national security.[1] The Civil Rights Movement and the Stonewall Riots further highlighted issues of inequity and safety across the United States and brought out engagement and demonstration across LGBTQ+ communities. The experience of many older gay and bisexual men living today, however, is perhaps most significantly marked by experiencing the HIV/acquired immunodeficiency syndrome

Pride at the Jefferson Center for Healthy Aging, Division of Geriatric Medicine and Palliative Care, Department of Family and Community Medicine, Thomas Jefferson University, 1015 Walnut Street, Suite 401, Philadelphia, PA 19147, USA
E-mail address: michael.danielewicz@jefferson.edu

Clin Geriatr Med 40 (2024) 239–250
https://doi.org/10.1016/j.cger.2023.11.003

(AIDS) epidemic firsthand starting in the 1980s. The impact it brought to their communities in particular continues to affect both those living with HIV and without in the form of survivor guilt, ongoing trauma, and intense experiences of loss.[2,3] The numbers by themselves are staggering: it is estimated that by 1995, one out of every nine gay men carried a diagnosis of AIDS. One out of fifteen had died of HIV/AIDS. Compounding the impact was a visible, public stigma of living—and dying—with the virus; the government itself was slow to acknowledge and respond to the crisis, with many framing it as a "morality" issue. As with many instances in LGBTQ+ history, it was direct action from within the communities that effected change.[4]

Today, well into the twenty-first century, the rights of potentially vulnerable LGBTQ+ individuals are again under threat from a variety of legislative efforts and social pressures across the United States. Even medicine itself has not always been receptive to the needs of gay and bisexual older men; access to equitable care has been historically limited and rife with potential for discrimination and stigmatization. Fortunately, this is changing as health care settings strive for inclusivity and as the body of research demonstrating unique community needs grows.

Older gay men have historically reported worse physical health compared with heterosexual older men, with higher rates of disability.[5] They have higher rates of alcohol and tobacco use and continue to be disproportionately affected by HIV.[6–8] Special considerations should be taken to screen for each of these unique aspects of health, as will be discussed.

Mental health disparities are also concerns for older gay and bisexual men: mental health issues have been reported to be more prevalent in these groups. Discrimination and stigma can cause and worsen such mental health issues, resulting in distress. Both gay and bisexual men may be subject to "double-discrimination:" discrimination and stigmatization that results from the intersection of multiple identities, in this case age and sexual orientation. Within gay and bisexual communities, which have tended to glorify youth and vitality, ageism (discrimination regarding age) has been a factor that can affect quality of life and make older community members feel alienated. Even so, connection to gay and bisexual communities can be powerful and give strength to older gay and bisexual men.[9] Older gay and bisexual individuals can provide important guidance and perspective to foster resiliency of their communities.

Older gay and bisexual adults can have unique caregiving needs. Research has shown that they are also more likely to live alone.[10] They may, given potential estrangement from biological families, rely on "families of choice"—informal caregiving networks they have built themselves. Even among those who are partnered, it was not until the same-sex marriage was legalized on a federal level that partners could take advantage of federal benefits; in some cases, this limited the ability of same-sex partners to act as surrogate decision-makers in medical emergencies.

Despite unique needs and vulnerabilities, research on LGBTQ+ older adults in general has been somewhat limited and largely focuses on limited samples of populations. Much work remains to be done to fully explore the unique needs of LGBTQ+ older adults. On the clinical front, LGBTQ+ older adults report experiencing health care that still operates with a lens of heterosexism (discrimination based on the assumption that heterosexuality is "normal").[11] Moving beyond this heteronormative framework has the potential to make all individuals feel welcome, accepted, and affirmed in health care settings. The result of this has been shown to go so far as to increase the likelihood of adherence to medical recommendations and treatments: one study has showed that those gay and bisexual male patients who disclose their sexual orientation to their providers are more likely to receive multiple appropriate health services, including vaccinations and sexually transmitted infection (STI) testing.[12]

Over many years, today's older gay and bisexual men have demonstrated resilience. Numerous studies have tried to capture this resilience—or even define it—with inconsistent results.[13] As the body of research develops and the health care climate changes and becomes more expansive, it is imperative that geriatric medicine physicians strive to create safe and inclusive spaces for older gay and bisexual men, in addition to other sexual and gender minorities (SGMs). One basic framework for this is summarized in **Table 1**, comprising both "cultural humility" and "medical competencies" (see also Noelle Marie Javier and Roy Noy's article, "Affirming Care for LGBTQ+ Patients," in this issue).

DISCUSSION

Mental Health

Multiple studies have shown that the prevalence of depression, suicide, and poor mental health is higher among LGB older adults compared with heterosexual counterparts.[14] Older gay and bisexual men face multiple unique challenges, including discrimination and stigma, social isolation, and concealment.

Discrimination and Stigma

Clinicians caring for older gay and bisexual men should be mindful of the mental health consequences of both recent and lifetime discrimination and stigma. The concept of dual stigma—being stigmatized for both age and sexual orientation—is particularly prescient and may affect mental health, especially as it intersects with other potentially-stigmatized identities. Many older gay and bisexual men have reported expectations and experiences of stigma and discrimination in health care settings. Such experiences, both recent and taken cumulatively over a lifetime, can predict psychological distress. Even within gay and bisexual communities, aging itself can be a stigmatizing condition, driving intra-community stigma. Given glamorization of youth and exclusion of older adults from focus, such "internalized gay ageism" can affect self-worth and create social stress as gay and bisexual men age. Even taken alone, internalized gay ageism has been shown to increase depressive symptoms.[15–17]

Concealment

Members of LGB communities may feel safer, affirmed, and more comfortable receiving care within their communities.[11] That said, given experiences and expectations of discrimination, some older gay and bisexual men may feel the need to conceal their sexual orientation in medical and mental health settings, making it more difficult to connect with physicians in an authentic way. Concealment has, given the lived experiences LGB older adults have, been a way of life for many to avoid discrimination,

Table 1
Selected components of affirming care for older gay and bisexual men

Cultural Humility	Medical Competency
Engagement in education on historical struggles with discrimination and stigma, in medicine and elsewhere	Familiarity with sexual health and screening needs
Language inclusive of same-sex partners	HIV management
Medical and sexual history inclusive of LGBTQIA+ identity and terminology	Identification of mental health concerns
Physical displays of inclusivity: flags, pins, and office décor	Screening for tobacco and alcohol use

even in health care.[11,16] It is essential for physicians and providers to create safe, affirming spaces where gay and bisexual men care share their identities and lived experiences to provide the best physical and mental health care.

Social Isolation and Loneliness

SAGE (Services and Advocacy for LGBT Elders) reports that LGBTQ+ individuals are twice as likely to be single and live alone and four times less likely to have children. Up to one-third to one-half of older bisexual men live alone, for example. This not only has implications on caregiving but may also affect connections to other individuals in general.[10,18] Not being in an intimate relationship and not being connected to gay communities has further been associated with increased loneliness in older gay men.[19] That said, a sizable Australian survey suggested that friendships and community support among older gay men provided significant support, highlighting the importance of so-called "families of choice."[20] Bisexual men and women may be at particular risk of poor mental health and loneliness given greater difficulty connecting to communities that are largely organized by and centered on gay men and lesbians.[14,21]

TOBACCO, ALCOHOL, AND SUBSTANCE USE

Physicians caring for gay and bisexual older men should be aware of the risks of tobacco, alcohol, and substance use within these communities.

Tobacco

The Centers for Disease Control (CDC) notes that gay men smoke at rates higher than the general population.[7] Data from the 2011 LGBT Health and Aging Report, which surveyed approximately 2500 LGBTQ+ older adults in the United States, suggested that 9% of gay men and 11% of bisexual men surveyed smoked.[6] Later analysis suggests that older gay and bisexual men have higher rates of smoking and excessive drinking compared with older lesbians and bisexual women.[22] A 2018 analysis revealed that older bisexual men had the highest prevalence of past-year smoking (51%) compared with gay and heterosexual counterparts. The same trend held true considering eligibility for low-dose CT screening for lung cancer based on history of tobacco use: 24.5% of bisexual men, compared with 9.1% of gay men and 15.2% of heterosexual people.[23] The implications of such data are broad, highlighting a need for targeted, tobacco use screening and intervention, in addition to offering appropriate lung cancer screening. Furthermore, specific data for older gay and bisexual men on electronic cigarette use are limited, warranting further investigation.

Alcohol

Alcohol may serve as a coping mechanism for victimization, marginalization, trauma, and discrimination. For older gay and bisexual men in particular, active instances of discrimination have been linked to alcohol consumption.[24] The LGBT Health and Aging report noted that 11% of gay men and 9% of bisexual men surveyed met criteria for "excessive" drinking: five or more alcoholic drinks per episode over the past 30 days.[6] In a 2017 cross-sectional survey of older LGB men and women, 22.4% of men surveyed met criteria for high-risk drinking, noting that increasing age was not linked to decreases in alcohol consumption, a trend unique to gay and bisexual men.[24]

Other Substances

It seems that older age may not be as much of a protective factor against substance use in LGB individuals as it is with heterosexual individuals.[25] The LGBT Health and

Aging report noted that 13% of gay men and 15% of bisexual men surveyed used non-prescribed drugs or substances.[6] In data collected from 2015 to 2017, 20.9% of older gay men and 20.4% of bisexual men reported drug use, compared with 10.2% of heterosexual men.[14] Some evidence suggests that substance use disorder is less prevalent in older LGB adults compared with younger individuals, but this field demands further research attention.[25] Social services and competent health care in general may be less available to LGBTQ+ older adults.[14] Compounding the issue is that little attention has been directed to the creation of programs for substance use disorder tailored to their unique needs.[21]

Exercise

Canadian data suggest that 11% of older men in the general population are engaging in recommended levels of physical activity.[26] This can have implications for both physical and mental health. Despite this low number, the 2011 Aging and Health Report reported that 82.4% of gay men and 82.1% of bisexual men surveyed reported "moderate" levels of physical activity, whereas 52.5% of gay men and 50.8% of bisexual men reported "vigorous" activity.[6] More recent data suggest that older gay men may be less physically active over the lifespan than heterosexual men, though the findings of studies are inconsistent on this matter.[27] Marginalization and discrimination of SGM people may limit community engagement related to exercise, as can heteronormativity in sports and organized exercise programs.[26,27] Connection to gay communities has been correlated with engagement in activities related to physical fitness. Such engagement may help combat some of the negative associations of aging and physical appearance within gay communities.[9] Research remains limited, however, as most data on physical activity come from younger men.[27] Further work may help elucidate the reasons older gay do or do not engage in physical activity. In clinic, connecting gay and bisexual older adults to leagues or clubs within LGBTQ+ communities could be beneficial not only in promoting exercise but also community engagement and resiliency.

Sexual Health

Recent analysis has suggested that LGB older adults are as likely as heterosexual older adults to remain sexually active as they age. That said, it is well-known within the medical community that less attention has been paid to the sexual needs and desires of older adults in general.[28] LGBTQ+ older adults are particularly vulnerable to unmet needs for acknowledgment of sexuality in addition to screening and counseling given that systems and structures are built with heterosexual relationships in mind. This can be particularly daunting in the realm of long-term care.[29]

In 2021, the National lesbian, gay, bisexual, transgender, queer, intersex, and asexual (LGBTQIA)+ Health Education Center and the National Center for Equitable Care for Elders offered suggestions for health care systems to ensure that care is inclusive of SGM people and their unique needs in sexual health. Per this guide, care for LGBTQ+ older adults begins long before contact with the medical professional. Check-in procedures should ask about gender identity and sexual orientation and signage should be inclusive, whereas promotional materials and practice décor should be inclusive of LGBTQ+ identities. The CDCs "five Ps" —partners, practices, past history of STIs, protection from STIs, and pregnancy—form the basis of a comprehensive sexual history. Additional "Ps" representing "pleasure" or "parts" have also been proposed.[29]

Currently, no specific guidelines for safer sex exist for older LGBTQ+ individuals outside the recommendations offered by national organizations for all age groups.[29]

It thus follows that the subsequent recommendations apply to older gay and bisexual men as well. The 2021 Centers for Disease Control guidelines recommend that sexually active men having sex with men be tested on an annual basis for gonorrhea and chlamydia at sites of sexual contact, with increased frequency based on risk. Potential sites of contact include the pharynx, urethra, and rectum. Of note, the guidelines recommend such testing irrespective of condom use. The CDC also recommends yearly testing for syphilis in all sexually active men who have sex with men (MSM), with increased frequency based on risk. Guidelines further recommend yearly HIV testing for sexually active men having sex with men if their HIV status is unknown or negative and the patient or their partner has had more than one partner because their last HIV screening.[30]

For those at high risk of HIV transmission, medications for preexposure prophylaxis (PrEP) can help mitigate HIV transmission risk. Potential bone density and renal function side effects are special considerations for older adults with some of these medications. PrEP is highly efficacious when taken daily and newer, long-acting injectable formulations may help facilitate adherence. Postexposure prophylaxis (PEP) for HIV can also be considered on a case-by-case basis for those who may have been exposed to the virus through sexual contact. Finally, PEP with doxycycline (doxy-PEP) is available a "morning-after pill" to reduce gonorrhea, chlamydia, and syphilis transmission by up to two-thirds; further research is still pending.[31] (Please also see Maile Young Karris and colleagues' article, "Preventive and Sexual Health in LGBTQ+ Older Adults," in this issue for an in-depth discussion.)

HIV in Gay and Bisexual Men

HIV has historically affected and continues to affect LGBTQ+ individuals disproportionately compared with non-SGM counterparts; this holds true into older age.[32] Among people living with HIV more than age 50 years, around 60% were gay or bisexual men as of 2015.[8] Even new HIV diagnoses tend to be skewing toward older demographics: according to the Centers for Disease Control's 2018 data more than 50% of new HIV diagnoses were in adults age 50 years and over. As of 2017, more than 50% of individuals living with HIV were also 50 years or older, showing HIV is now largely a chronic disease of older adults.[33]

The historical background of HIV in older gay and bisexual male communities is, as has already been covered, complex. Some gay and bisexual men with HIV today likely did not expect to survive to older adulthood. In one study, 20% of individuals surveyed reported losing 15 or more friends to HIV during the height of the AIDS epidemic during the 1980s and 1990s.[15] Throughout this history, some older gay and bisexual men may feel—or even experience—that being both gay and HIV positive had a negative effect on their experiences with health care providers.[34] As geriatric medicine places increasing emphasis on how older adults can experience "healthy aging," it becomes increasingly important to understand the history and lived experiences of those with HIV, as well as ongoing disparities.[35]

Those living with HIV often experience multiple other comorbidities, polypharmacy, and physical/cognitive changes.[36] Gay and bisexual men with HIV are more likely to experience worse health status, higher number of chronic conditions, anxiety, and depression compared with those without HIV. Many of these disparities based on historical as well as psychosocial and biological roots help explain the worse health status reported by older gay and bisexual adults living with HIV, creating a "within-group" marginalization compared with those not living with HIV.[36] It is critically important that physicians focus on providing additional support and services to older gay and bisexual men living with HIV to promote physical and mental well-being.

CANCER RISK AND SCREENING

Disparities in cancer and cancer screening are less well-studied in LGBTQ+ older adults compared with other health measures such as tobacco use. Part of this is due to the reality that collection of sexual orientation and gender identity (SOGI) data in oncology has been limited. Some cancer epidemiology related to SOGI has been extrapolated by locations with higher concentrations of SGM individuals. Some of this extrapolated data has, for instance, suggested that prostate cancer rates in gay men may be lower than heterosexual counterparts, though this is far from a certain conclusion. Similarly, geographic areas with a higher density of bisexual men have been suggested to have higher incidence of colorectal cancer. This conclusion has also been called into question. Cancers related to viral etiologies (HIV, HPV, hepatitis) as well as modifiable health behaviors (smoking, alcohol use) have become a particular focus of cancer prevention efforts in gay and bisexual men.[37,38] Studies analyzing cancer screening in gay and bisexual men are similarly limited.[39]

Prostate Cancer

A 2008 report from California Health Interview Survey (CHIS) data suggested that gay/bisexual men had lower odds of undergoing prostate-specific antigen (PSA) testing as a screening for prostate cancer compared with heterosexual individuals.[40] A more recent evaluation based on data from the National Health Interview Survey for 2013, 2015, and 2018 found that compared with heterosexual men, gay men being screened for prostate cancer were younger (median age 58 vs 64). They were also more likely to have discussed PSA testing with their physicians and providers. That said, by 2018, rates of completing screening were no different between gay and heterosexual men. Of note, the age of screening and rates of screening for bisexual men were closer to the heterosexual population in this study.[41]

Colorectal Cancer

The 2008 CHIS analysis found that gay/bisexual men were significantly more likely to undergo screening for colorectal cancer.[40] A study using data from the 2016 Behavioral Risk Factor Surveillance System also found higher rates of colorectal cancer screening among lesbian and gay individuals (74.1%) compared with heterosexual (68.5%) and bisexual (68.2%) individuals. These differences were not significant when controlling for other variables. The investigators concluded that sociodemographic characteristics were more likely responsible for differing screening rates for colorectal cancer.[42]

Anal Cancer

Anal cancer screening has been a particular area of both interest and controversy. Men living with HIV and gay/bisexual men have a higher rate of anal human papillomavirus (HPV) infection than other populations, which can predispose to anal dysplasia and anal cancer.[43]

In 2022, the prospective randomized control ANal Cancer/HSIL Outcomes Research (ANCHOR) study demonstrated that screening individuals with HIV with cytology and treating precancerous changes decreased the risk of progression to anal cancer by 57%.[44] Anal cytology is performed via the use of a moistened swab inserted 4 to 6 cm into the anal canal and removed under firm rotating circumferential pressure, which is then placed into the same medium used for Pap testing. Unlike cervical cancer screening, there are no widely accepted guidelines for result interpretation and action plan.[45] Currently, no national guideline exists that recommends screening for anorectal cancer with anal cytology.

The New York State AIDS Institute has promulgated a series of recommendations for screening for anal and perianal dysplasia, though its recommendations are limited to individuals with HIV. There remain no widely accepted recommendations for anal cancer screening in gay and bisexual men of any age in the absence of HIV.

The New York State guidelines recommend, for all patients more than 35 years with HIV, that physicians and providers annually do the following.

- Inquire about anorectal symptoms including itching, bleeding, masses, pain, tenesmus, and rectal fullness
- Visually inspect an area within a 5 cm radius of the anal verge
- Discuss screening for rectal cancer
  - Considering cytology before digital rectal examination
- Perform digital rectal examination annually or at any time in the presence of symptoms

For individuals living with HIV who are MSM (MSM), transgender men, or transgender women, New York State recommends annually performing anal cytology, also known as "anal pap."

In the presence of low-grade squamous intraepithelial lesion (LSIL) or high-grade squamous intraepithelial lesion (HSIL) findings on cytology, these guidelines recommend high-resolution anoscopy and biopsy. For atypical squamous cells of undetermined significance (ASC-US) results, HPV testing is indicated. Negative HPV testing warrants repeat cytology in 1 year, whereas positive HPV testing warrants high-resolution anoscopy.

Per the New York State guidelines, and particularly salient to geriatric medicine, providers may consider discontinuing anal cancer screening when the patient life expectancy is thought to be less than 10 years or if an individual is not sexually active and two consecutive cytology results have returned negative.[43]

Recommendations for anal cancer screening in gay and bisexual men who do not have HIV have proven more controversial; significant differences in practice continue to exist. Currently, most gay and bisexual men without HIV do not receive routine anal cancer screening.[46] Despite this, multiple studies have shown than gay men and bisexual men are more likely to undergo anal cancer screening than heterosexual men.[39] Many gay men and bisexual men are interested and may consider screening for anal cancer if offered.[47]

A 2021 review provided recommendations for consideration of anal cancer prevention in MSM who do not have HIV, noting that guidelines remain elusive in the setting of limited data. Specifically, the investigators note consideration of HPV vaccination in gay and bisexual men more than age 45 years. Although currently not part of either Centers for Disease Control or Food and Drug Administration recommendations, the investigators state that the clear efficacy of the vaccine in protecting against HPV before exposure could offer some protection. The investigators further note that digital rectal examination alone may not identify high-risk HSIL lesions as they are frequently not readily palpable.[46]

Currently, most screening algorithms are based on local practice and expert opinion. Digital rectal examination should be performed in all patients with symptoms concerning for anorectal cancer, though this recommendation is also based largely off expert opinion and cohort studies.[45] Further study and extrapolation of results from the ANCHOR study may help provide clearer recommendations and guidelines for anal cancer screening in individuals without HIV. For the time being, physicians should rely on informed discussions with patients, including discussion of the risks (discomfort, false positive cytology and resulting anxiety/further testing) and potential benefits (early identification of precancerous lesions).[43]

SUMMARY

Older gay and bisexual men have long experienced discrimination and stigma. Part of their lived experiences may help explain higher rates of medical and mental health concerns. Mental health issues and psychological distress have been reported to be more prevalent in older gay and bisexual men, as has worse self-reported overall health. HIV in particular has disproportionally affected older gay and bisexual men, some of whom survived the initial outbreak of the epidemic in the 1980s and 1990s. Physicians and providers should be mindful of the need to adequately screen gay and bisexual older adults for psychological trauma, tobacco and alcohol use, and sexually transmitted infections, in addition to routine screenings for cancer. Creation of safe and affirming spaces for medical care—inclusive of lived experiences of older gay and bisexual men—can help create truly inclusive environments and improve health care participation and outcomes.

CLINICS CARE POINTS

- Inclusive language and medical interviewing can create safe, equitable, affirming spaces for care.
- Gay and bisexual older men face stigma from the general population, health care, and within their own LGBTQ+ communities that has shaped their experiences and, in many instances, physical and mental health.
- Physicians should screen gay and bisexual older men for alcohol, tobacco, and other substance use.
- Sexual history should be inclusive of LGBTQ+ identities and experiences.
- The Centers for Disease Control recommends routine screening for sexually-transmitted infections in sexually active gay and bisexual males, including older adults.
- HIV continues to disproportionately affect gay and bisexual men; demographics show that both incidence and prevalence of those living with HIV are trending older.
- Anal cancer screening for gay and bisexual men remains controversial; guidelines currently available recommends screening individuals with HIV more than age 35 years and considering discontinuing screening when life expectancy is thought to be less than 10 years.

DISCLOSURE

No disclosures.

REFERENCES

1. Adkins J. "These people are frightened to death:" congressional investigations and the lavender Scare. National Archives Prologue Magazine 2016;48(2).
2. Sichel A. "I knew these marvelous people": gay men's experiences of long-term HIV/AIDS survival long-term HIV/AIDS survival. Dissertation. City University of New York, 2022.

3. Odets W. In the shadow of the epidemic:being HIV-negative in the age of AIDS. Duke University Press; 1995.
4. Rosenfeld D. The AIDS epidemic's lasting impact on gay men. The British Academy; 2018.
5. Fredriksen-Goldsen KI, Kim HJ, Barkan SE, et al. Health disparities among lesbian, gay, and bisexual older adults: results from a population-based study. Am J Publ Health 2013;103(10):1802–9.
6. Fredriksen-Goldsen KI, Kim H, Emlet CA, et al. The aging and health report: disparities and resilience among lesbian, gay, bisexual, and transgender older adults. Institute for Multigenerational Health; 2011.
7. Gay and Bisexual Men's Health. Smoking & tobacco use. Centers for Disease Control and Prevention; 2016.
8. Brennan-Ing M. Caregiving for aging LGBT adults with HIV. American Psychological Association; 2015.
9. Brennan-Ing M, Haberlen S, Ware D, et al. Psychological connection to the gay community and negative self-appraisals in middle-aged and older men who have sex with men: the mediating effects of fitness engagement. J Gerontol B Psychol Sci Soc Sci 2022;77(1):39–49.
10. Fredriksen-Goldsen KI, Hoy-Ellis CP, Goldsen J, et al. Creating a vision for the future: key competencies and strategies for culturally competent practice with lesbian, gay, bisexual, and transgender (LGBT) older adults in the health and human services. J Gerontol Soc Work 2014;57(2–4):80–107. https://doi.org/10.1080/01634372.2014.890690.
11. Choi SK, Meyer IH. LGBT+ aging: a review of research findings, needs, and policy implications. The Williams Institute; 2016. UCLA School of Law.
12. Petroll AE, Mosack KE. Physician awareness of sexual orientation and preventive health recommendations to men who have sex with men. Sex Transm Dis 2011; 38(1):63–7. https://doi.org/10.1097/OLQ.0b013e3181ebd50f.
13. Jurček A, Keogh B, Sheaf G, et al. Defining and researching the concept of resilience in LGBT+ later life: findings from a mixed study systematic review. PLoS One 2022;17(11):e0277384.
14. Han BH, Duncan DT, Arcila-Mesa M, et al. Co-occurring mental illness, drug use, and medical multimorbidity among lesbian, gay, and bisexual middle-aged and older adults in the United States: a nationally representative study. BMC Publ Health 2020;20(1):1123.
15. Wight RG, LeBlanc AJ, de Vries B, et al. Stress and mental health among midlife and older gay-identified men. Am J Publ Health 2012;102(3):503–10.
16. Kia H, Salway T, Lacombe-Duncan A, et al. "You could tell I said the wrong things": constructions of sexual identity among older gay men in healthcare settings. Qual Health Res 2022;32(2):255–66.
17. Wight RG, LeBlanc AJ, Meyer IH, et al. Internalized gay ageism, mattering, and depressive symptoms among midlife and older gay-identified men. Soc Sci Med 2015;147:200–8.
18. Facts on LGBT Aging. SAGE and the national resource center on LGBT aging 2021.
19. Hughes M, Lyons A, Alba B, et al. Predictors of loneliness among older lesbian and gay people. J Homosex 2023;70(5):917–37.
20. Lyons A, Pitts M, Grierson J. Growing old as a gay man: psychosocial well-being of a sexual minority. Res Aging 2013;35(3):275–95.
21. Yarns BC, Abrams JM, Meeks TW, et al. The mental health of older LGBT adults. Curr Psychiatr Rep 2016;18(6):60.

22. Fredriksen-Goldsen KI, Emlet CA, Kim HJ, et al. The physical and mental health of lesbian, gay male, and bisexual (LGB) older adults: the role of key health indicators and risk and protective factors. Gerontol 2013;53(4):664–75.
23. Matthews AK, McCabe SE, Lee JGL, et al. Differences in smoking prevalence and eligibility for low-dose computed tomography (LDCT) lung cancer screening among older U.S. adults: role of sexual orientation. Cancer Causes Control 2018; 29(8):769–74.
24. Bryan AE, Kim HJ, Fredriksen-Goldsen KI. Factors associated with high-risk alcohol consumption among LGB older adults: the roles of gender, social support, perceived stress, discrimination, and stigma. Gerontol 2017;57(suppl 1): S95–104.
25. Green KE, Feinstein BA. Substance use in lesbian, gay, and bisexual populations: an update on empirical research and implications for treatment. Psychol Addict Behav 2012;26(2):265–78.
26. Thandi MKG, Phinney A, Oliffe JL, et al. Engaging older men in physical activity: implications for health promotion practice. Am J Men's Health 2018;12(6): 2064–75.
27. Kendrick D, Hughes M, Coutts R, et al. Older gay men's engagement with physical activity: a scoping review. Health Soc Care Community 2021;29(6):e457–66.
28. Brennan-Ing M, Kaufman JE, Larson B, et al. Sexual health among lesbian, gay, bisexual, and heterosexual older adults: an exploratory analysis. Clin Gerontol 2021;44(3):222–34.
29. Ard KL, Mather A, Riedy CA. Sexual health care for older LGBTQIA+ older adults. National LGBTQIA+ Health Education Center and National Center for Equitable Care for Elders; 2021.
30. Sexually transmitted infections treatment guidelines. Centers for Disease Control and Prevention; 2021.
31. Traeger MW, Mayer KH, Krakower DS, et al. Potential impact of doxycycline post-exposure prophylaxis prescribing strategies on incidence of bacterial sexually transmitted infections. Clin Infect Dis 2023;ciad488. https://doi.org/10.1093/cid/ciad488.
32. HIV/AIDS. Sage. 2023.
33. HIV and specific populations. National Institutes of Health; 2021.
34. Singleton MC, Green DC, Enguidanos SM. Identifying healthcare stereotype threat in older gay men living with HIV. J Appl Gerontol 2023;42(9):1965–73. https://doi.org/10.1177/07334648231167944.
35. Emlet CA, Shiu C, Kim HJ, et al. Bouncing back: resilience and mastery among HIV-positive older gay and bisexual men. Gerontol 2017;57(suppl 1):S40–9.
36. Older people living with HIV. SAGE; 2019.
37. Emlet CA, Fredriksen-Goldsen KI, Kim HJ, et al. Accounting for HIV health disparities: risk and protective factors among older gay and bisexual men. J Aging Health 2020;32(7–8):677–87.
38. Cathcart-Rake EJ. Cancer in sexual and gender minority patients: are we addressing their needs? Curr Oncol Rep 2018;20(11):85.
39. Heer E, Peters C, Knight R, et al. Participation, barriers, and facilitators of cancer screening among LGBTQ+ populations: a review of the literature. Prev Med 2023;170:107478. https://doi.org/10.1016/j.ypmed.2023.107478.
40. Heslin KC, Gore JL, King WD, et al. Sexual orientation and testing for prostate and colorectal cancers among men in California. Med Care 2008;46(12):1240–8.
41. Wilcox Vanden Berg RN, Basourakos SP, Shoag J, et al. Prostate cancer screening for gay men in the United States. Urology 2022;163:119–25.

42. Charkhchi P, Schabath MB, Carlos RC. Modifiers of cancer screening prevention among sexual and gender minorities in the behavioral risk factor surveillance system. J Am Coll Radiol 2019;16(4 Pt B):607–20.
43. Hirsch BE, McGowan JP, Fine SM, et al. Screening for anal dysplasia and cancer in adults with HIV. Johns Hopkins University; 2022.
44. Palefsky JM, Lee JY, Jay N, et al. Treatment of anal high-grade squamous intraepithelial lesions to prevent anal cancer. N Engl J Med 2022;386(24):2273–82.
45. Barroso LF, Stier EA, Hillman R, et al. Anal cancer screening and prevention: summary of evidence reviewed for the 2021 Centers for disease control and prevention sexually transmitted infection guidelines. Clin Infect Dis 2022;74(Suppl_2): S179–92.
46. Fuchs MA, Multani AG, Mayer KH, et al. Anal cancer screening for HIV-negative men who have sex with men: making clinical decisions with limited data. LGBT Health 2021;8(5):317–21.
47. Schofield AM, Sadler L, Nelson L, et al. A prospective study of anal cancer screening in HIV-positive and negative MSM. AIDS 2016;30(9):1375–83.

Medical Issues Affecting Older Lesbian and Bisexual Women

Angela D. Primbas, MD[a,*], Al Ogawa, MD[b]

KEYWORDS

- Lesbian • Bisexual • Older adults • Geriatrics • Health disparities • LGBTQIA+

KEY POINTS

- Characterize and historically contextualize the unique health experiences of older lesbian and bisexual women within the broader lesbian, gay, bisexual, transgender, queer or questioning, or another diverse gender identity (LGBTQ+) community.
- Identify the social factors that impact healthy aging among lesbian and bisexual women including the compounding effect of lifelong discrimination.
- Recognize gaps in the literature regarding lesbian and bisexual aging, and propose opportunities for targeted research.

INTRODUCTION

The existing research on the lesbian, gay, bisexual, transgender, queer or questioning, or another diverse gender identity (LGBTQ+) community inadequately depicts lesbian and bisexual (LB) women's experiences in comparison to that of gay men or transgender/gender-diverse individuals.[1] Older LB women have even less representation in the academic literature compared to younger women. However, the existing research demonstrates both resilience and compounding effects of lifelong discrimination on overall health, disability, and resources.

HISTORY

LB women were often excluded from these social movements. For example, leaders of the women's movement purposefully distanced themselves from issues impacting lesbian, bisexual, and transgender women, especially those with intersectional identities, believing that including these populations would hamper their ability to create

[a] Division of Geriatrics, Department of Medicine, UCLA David Geffen School of Medicine, University of California, 200 Medical Plaza, Suite 365A, Los Angeles, CA 90024, USA; [b] Swedish Cherry Hill Family Medicine Residency
* Corresponding author.
E-mail address: aprimbas@mednet.ucla.edu

Clin Geriatr Med 40 (2024) 251–260
https://doi.org/10.1016/j.cger.2023.12.001

social change. Lesbian women were dubbed "the lavender menace" by leaders of the women's movement, a term that was later reclaimed by lesbian feminist activists.[2,3]

LB women have distinct experiences and associated trauma that directly relate to oppressive policies and sociocultural climates of their time. LB women were often pivotal leaders of social change throughout history yet were often excluded from the benefits their work for social movements garnered. As a result, the experience of aging for LB women within each of these generations accompanies different associated risks, resources, and resilience.[3]

Even within communities of LB women, experiences vary significantly. Age, race, class, disability, education, religion, and citizenship status (among numerous other factors) come together to impact each person's lived experience. Yet an intersectional and nuanced research lens is often lacking. LB women are often grouped together in studies, and transgender women's identities are excluded, despite each group facing distinct challenges and disparities. Bisexual women are at higher risk of adverse health, economic, and social outcomes compared to almost every other subgroup in the LGBTQ+ community.[4] Transgender women are variably excluded or obscured in research about LGBTQ+ women. Finally, black, indigenous, (and) people of color (BIPOC) LB women's experiences are often othered or omitted.

GENERAL HEALTH AND PREVENTATIVE CARE

Studies have found that LB women are less likely to have consistent access to health services than heterosexual women. A 2011 Institute of Medicine report demonstrated that LB women seek health care less frequently, are less likely to receive preventative health care, and have lower adherence rates for prescribed treatment protocols than their heterosexual counterparts. In another study, LB women were less likely to have health insurance and more likely to face financial difficulties with health-related costs than heterosexual women.[3] A survey of older lesbian, gay, and bisexual (LGB) adults in California found that older LB women were at risk of delayed access to care.[5,6]

Accessing safe and consistent care is also related to feeling comfortable with providers, empowering providers to provide appropriate care. Over 1 in 10 lesbian women and 1 in 3 bisexual women have not disclosed their orientation to any health provider, and research suggests that LB women who have not disclosed their identities are less likely to seek regular health care.[7] In a national sample of older LB women, 35% of lesbians and 35% of bisexual women reported being very or somewhat concerned that the quality of care they would receive would be adversely impacted by their sexual orientation.[8] Evidence from focus groups suggests that LB women pay attention to the affirming cues in the health care setting (ie, language on forms, LGBTQ+-friendly materials, and so forth) as well as the provider interaction when deciding about identity disclosure.[9,10]

Multiple studies have documented lower rates of routine cancer screening including mammography and Papanicolaou (Pap) tests among LB women.[3,4] Negative prior experiences with the health care system and mistrust of health care providers contribute to these lower rates of engagement.[11] The few studies that do examine older LB women find that this persists in later life.[6]

There are differences even between LB women, as in almost every available study bisexual women are described as less likely to engage in regular health care visits, have more financial barriers to care, and are more likely to describe being in worse overall health compared to lesbian women.[3] LB women are often grouped together as a monolith but have different experiences and health risk factors.

CARDIOVASCULAR DISEASE AND RISK FACTORS

Studies are mixed when describing rates of cardiovascular risk factors and disease among older LB women. Several longitudinal studies have shown that LB women develop higher rates of cardiovascular risk factors including obesity, hypertension, and type II diabetes compared to heterosexual women, with equivocal data regarding frank cardiovascular disease.[3,4,12,13] Fredriksen and colleagues found that heightened risks of cardiovascular disease among LB women emerge later in life, and it is likely that risk factor disparities earlier in life (smoking, obesity) influence disparities in cardiovascular disease later in life.[5] In these studies, bisexual women had a higher prevalence of almost all risk factors when compared to lesbian women.

A May 2023 study found that LB women had lower Life's Essential 8 scores (a measure of cardiovascular health that involves body mass index, blood glucose and lipid levels, and health behaviors) compared to their heterosexual counterparts.[14]

Evidence is conflicting on diet and physical activity—some studies have demonstrated no difference between rates of physical activity among LB women,[12,15] while others indicated lower rates.[16] Most studies indicate no difference in dietary practices.[17] Almost all studies (while limited in number) identify worse overall health (especially subjectively) among older LB women compared to heterosexual women, despite mixed data on physical disease prevalence.[6]

MENTAL HEALTH

LB women's mental health and the impact of minority stress and compounded trauma have been comparatively better studied. Studies have found that LB women have higher rates of depression, anxiety, and post-traumatic stress disorder compared to heterosexual women.[15] In a 2021 to 2022 national survey, LB women had higher rates of all mental health conditions, including major depressive disorder and suicidal ideation, when compared to heterosexual women. Again, there was a trend that bisexual women had higher rates of mental health disorders compared to lesbian women.[18] Higher rates of depression among LB women are present across all ages—older LB women continue to have higher rates of depression compared to heterosexual women.[19] Several studies indicate that these trends continue later in life.[6] The Aging and Health Report found that 35% of older bisexual women experienced depression compared to 27% of older lesbian women.[20]

The social contexts that many LGBTQ+ older adults have lived through have exposed this population to multiple types of victimization and discrimination.[3] Research consistently demonstrates that early life events have profound impact on later life stages, and perceived discrimination, internalized stigma, identity concealment, and victimization may have profound mental health consequences.[21]

In particular, older bisexual individuals have higher levels of internalized stigma and sexual identity concealment and subsequently higher risk of mental health disorders compared to older lesbian and gay populations, which may intersect with discrimination based on BIPOC status.[19]

ALCOHOL AND SMOKING

Research suggests LB women are more likely to smoke cigarettes at younger and older ages compared to heterosexual women despite decreasing smoking rates with age.[3,22] Fredriksen-Goldsen and colleagues[3] found that 18% of older LB women smoked compared to 11% of older heterosexual women.

LB women are also more likely to engage in binge drinking and meet criteria for alcohol use disorder compared to heterosexual women.[10,23] Rowan and colleagues[24] found that older LB women were significantly more likely to report alcohol use disorders, substance use disorders, and smoking compared to older heterosexual women. Rates of illicit substance use (including chronic opioid use) are also higher among LB women.[25]

Within the LB population, bisexual women have higher rates of alcohol and substance use. Bisexual women have been found to have higher rates of smoking, substance use, hazardous drinking, symptoms of dependence, and binge drinking compared to lesbian women.[25,26]

Experiences of minority stress are also thought to contribute to higher rates of alcohol, smoking, and substance use among LB women. This theory postulates that chronic social stress related to prejudice and discrimination (both interpersonal and institutionalized) contributes to psychological distress and substance use as a possible coping mechanism.[27]

Theories behind the uniquely high substance use risk among bisexual women include the cultural invisibility of bisexuality as well as associated stigma.[28] Bisexual individuals experience stigma from both heterosexual populations as well as gay men and lesbian women, often being characterized as being confused or lying about their identity as they do not adhere to a binary model of sexual orientation.[29] Even many LGBTQ+ populations have little focus or resources for bisexual individuals (despite evidence that the community makes up about 70% of the broader LGBTQ+ population).[30] This lower visibility and lack of connectedness from both the heterosexual population and the LGBTQ+ community is thought to contribute to higher levels of internalized stigma and mental distress and, subsequently, higher rates of substance use.[31]

CANCER SCREENING

As previously alluded to, LB women are at higher risk for behavioral risk factors associated with certain types of cancers compared to heterosexual women. LB women have higher rates of alcohol use and smoking as discussed, as well as higher rates of nulliparity and lower use of oral contraceptives which can be protective against gynecologic and breast cancers.[32]

Despite increased associated risks, LB women are less likely to undergo routine cancer screening, mirroring lower primary care engagement. Lesbian women, in particular, are less likely to undergo Pap screening compared to heterosexual women, likely reflecting the misconception that lesbian women do not need the same cervical cancer screening as heterosexual women.[32,33] LB women are as likely as heterosexual women to get cervical cancer but are up to 10 times less likely to undergo screening.[33] A majority of studies demonstrate consistently that LB women have lower rates of cervical cancer screening compared to heterosexual women.[32,34,35]

Regarding breast cancer screening, 1 study found that lesbian women were less likely than heterosexual women to have ever had a mammogram across all age groups (including older populations), which has been corroborated in older LB populations.[3,32] With regard to colonoscopies, LB women have lower rates of recommended screening adherence compared to heterosexual women.[36]

While several studies have documented lower screening rates for LB women, data on prevalence of different cancers among older LB women are mixed or insufficient.[37] It is commonly cited that LB women may be at higher risk for breast, cervical, and ovarian cancer, but more research is needed.[34]

DISABILITY

LB women overall report high rates of disability and higher rates compared to heterosexual women.[3,19] In a national study assessing disparities among LGBTQ+ older adults, 47% of LGBTQ+ older adults reported being disabled, including 53% of lesbian women and 51% of bisexual women.[20] When compared with heterosexual women, older LB women had higher rates of disability (44% to 36% in another study).[3,6] Some argue that these increased disability rates are influenced, at least in part, by life perspectives from cumulative experiences of discrimination and victimization during eras of stigmatization, criminalization, and social erasure of same-sex identities.[3]

MEMORY AND COGNITION

Theories suggest that minority stress over a lifetime heightens the risk of premature cognitive aging and decline among LGBTQ+ older adults.[38] According to the Alzheimer's Association, approximately 350,000 LGBTQ+ older adults are currently living with cognitive impairment, and 7.4% of the LGB population over 50 is living with dementia.[39,40]

Few studies investigate the risk of cognitive impairment among older LGBTQ+ populations. Some have found higher risk of cognitive decline among LGBTQ+ people compared to heterosexual counterparts,[41] but data are often mixed.[42]

There is little research on cognition of older LB women, but 1 study did find that older bisexual women had higher odds of reporting difficulty concentrating, remembering, or making decisions than older heterosexual women, but it found no difference between lesbian and heterosexual women.[43] Other studies have found no difference in self-rated memory between LGB older adults and heterosexual peers.[44,45]

SOCIAL FACTORS THAT IMPACT HEALTHY AGING

Healthy aging is not only characterized by timely and consistent access to medical resources but is also dramatically impacted by social and economic forces that shape overall quality of life. LGBTQ+ elders face a series of barriers that impact their ability to achieve social and economic stability, and as a result, they are more vulnerable to insecurity as they age than their heterosexual peers. At the same time, LGBTQ+ older adults demonstrate remarkable resilience in the face of a lifetime of discrimination and form strong community bonds and supports, including families of choice.

Experiences of Discrimination

Trauma from repeated experiences with discrimination has a compounding effect over a lifetime. In the Aging and Health Report, 68% of LGBTQ+ older adults surveyed reported experiencing verbal insults related to their gender or sexual identity, while 43% experienced direct threats of physical violence (20% were victims of physical assault).[20]

During older LB adults' lifetimes, existing as oneself came with high risks of physical threats and violence, not to mention discrimination in employment, housing, and benefits. Looking at experiences of trauma by generation—LGBTQ+ adults aged 80 and above (Greatest Generation and the Silent Generation) have the highest rates of internalized stigma and identity concealment but are individually less likely to have experienced discrimination and victimization, suggesting concealment may have been protective. Members of the younger Pride Generation have lower rates of internalized stigma and identity concealment but have higher rates of discrimination, victimization, loneliness, and social isolation.[2] These perspectives are important to consider, as disparities in health and social resources may differ by generation based on trauma experience.

Housing and Benefits

Concerns about housing discrimination is prevalent in the LGBTQ+ community, with 73% of respondents in a national study reporting concerns with either renting or buying a home. In 2014, approximately 48% of LGB couples attempting to rent a home experienced at least 1 form of adverse treatment based on their sexual orientation.[46] LGBTQ+ seniors face further concerns when looking specifically for senior housing communities—according to 1 study, only 18% of senior housing communities had policies that prohibit discrimination based on gender or sexual identity in 2021.[47]

Finances, Spousal Benefits, and Economic Stability

LB older women face economic and financial insecurity as their ability to build wealth has been impacted by a lifetime of employment discrimination and a lack of legal recognition to acquire partner benefits.[20,47]

Due at least in part to these challenges in building wealth, LGBTQ+ older people are more likely to live at or below 200% of the federal poverty level compared to heterosexual people (33% compared to 25%, respectively). Rates are especially high among bisexual older women, with 48% living at or below 200% of the federal poverty line (the same rate as transgender older adults).[8,48] The Institute of Medicine report found that lesbian couples, in particular, had lower income levels than comparably aged heterosexual couples "likely owing to employment discrimination over their lifetimes and the concomitant earnings disparities, reduced lifelong earnings, lower social security payments, and fewer opportunities to build pensions."[23]

Social Isolation, Social Support, Caregiving, and Long-Term Care

LGBTQ+ older adults are more likely to live alone and more likely to report being lonely than their heterosexual peers. Many LGBTQ+ older adults have built strong networks of friends and chosen family as a form of resilience after rejection or disownment from biological families.[8,49]

Despite this connection, many older LB women live alone compared to their heterosexual counterparts. 39% of older lesbian women and 48% of older bisexual women are unpartnered.[8] LB women have particularly robust social networks compared to other LGBTQ+ older adults. Older bisexual women have larger social networks than their lesbian or gay counterparts.[4,49]

Biological family disconnection and homophobic adoptions policies render LGBTQ+ older adults less likely to have relatives or biological, formally recognized children able to assist with caregiving.[8,48] As a result, there is greater reliance on chosen family and care webs for caregiving needs, which can be hard when these chosen families are also aging. About 83% of lesbian and 76% bisexual women are concerned about adequate caregiving and social support as they age.[48,49]

Loss of independence and increased care dependence can be particularly challenging and traumatic for LB women, who often have additional concerns related to senior housing and long-term care facility access. The most cited concern for LB women is "going back into the closet" in order to receive nondiscriminatory long-term care and resources.[50]

Resiliency

Despite life-long experiences with inequity and discrimination, LGBTQ+ older adults have proven to be remarkably resilient—research consistently demonstrates that

LGBTQ+ older adults form strong communities and bonds and provide each other with support that society often denied.[20] LB leaders, in particular, have been integral to numerous social movements, fostering community, change, and survival amidst discrimination.

SUMMARY

LB women face increased barriers to accessing care due to fears of discrimination and poor prior experiences with health providers. LB women are more likely to have chronic medical conditions and disability later in life, as well as suffer higher levels of mental distress. Bisexual women, in particular, face heightened risks of lack of engagement in primary care and screening, mental health disorders, and substance use.

Historical context and an intersectional lens are important in understanding the experiences of older LB women and the challenges that they face. The oldest generations may not experience as much overt discrimination due to high rates of identity concealment as a protective mechanism in a hostile society. Discriminatory policies across a lifetime have resulted in LB women having less financial resources as they age. LB women have renewed concerns of discrimination and mistreatment in aging as they require more assistance and caregiving. Despite these challenges, LB women form strong social networks and communities and compensate for some lacking resources through mutual support.

While there is a growing field of research in LGBTQ+ health, most studies are small and community based. It proves challenging to encompass the diverse arrays of aging experiences within the existing literature. Dedicated research on the experiences and health of older LB women is sorely needed to help support this population in aging.

CLINICS CARE POINTS AND RECOMMENDATIONS

- LB women are a growing and understudied population among older adults.
- Older LB women have higher risk of diabetes, hypertension, obesity, disability, depression, and substance use compared to heterosexual women.
- Older LB women are less likely to engage in preventative care and screening than heterosexual women and have concerns about mistreatment by health providers.
- Lifetimes of discrimination and unequal policies result in compounded trauma and fewer material and social resources later in life.
- Older bisexual women, in particular, are at comparatively high risk of several medical issues.
- Providers should be attuned to historical and current challenges in accessing accepting and comprehensive health care.

DISCLOSURE

Neither author has any relationships or affiliations to disclose.

REFERENCES

1. Fredriksen-Goldsen K, Kim HJ. The science of conducting research with LGBT older adults – an introduction to aging with Pride: national health, aging and Sexuality/gender study (NHAS). Gerontol 2017;57(suppl 1):S1–4.

2. Fredriksen-Goldsen K. The Future of LGBT+ aging: a Blueprint for action in services, policies, and research. Generations 2016;40(2):6–15.
3. Fredriksen-Goldsen K, Kim H, Barkan S, et al. Health Disparities among lesbian, gay and bisexual older adults: results from a population based study. Am J Public Health 2013;103(10):1802–9.
4. Fredriksen-Goldsen KI, Shiu C, Bryan AEB, et al. Health equity and aging of bisexual older adults: pathways of risk and resilience. The Journal of Gerontology Series B: Psychological Sciences and Social Sciences 2016. https://doi.org/10.1093/geronb/gbw120. gbw120.
5. Institute of Medicine Committee on Lesbian. Gay, bisexual and transgender health issues and research gaps and opportunities; board on the health of Select populations. The health of lesbian, gay, bisexual and transgender (LGBT) people: building a Foundation of better understanding. Washington D.C.: National Academies Press; 2011.
6. Wallace SP, Cochran SD, Durazo EM, et al. The health of aging lesbian, gay and bisexual adults in California. Los Angeles: University of California, Los Angeles Center for Health Policy Research; 2011.
7. McNair RP, Hegarty K, Taft A. Disclosure for same-sex attracted women enhancing the quality of the patient-doctor relationship in general practice. Soc Sci Med 2015; 75:208–16.
8. AARP Research. Maintaining Dignity: understanding and responding to the challenges facing older LGBT Americans. Washington, D.C. 2018 https://doi.org/10.26419/res.00217.001.
9. Fredericks E, Harbin A, Baker K. Being (in)visible in the clinic: a qualitative study of queer, lesbian and bisexual women's health care experiences in Eastern Canada. Health Care Women Int 2016;38:394–408.
10. Grella CE, Greenwell L, Mays VM, et al. Influence of gender, sexual orientation and need on treatment utilization for substance use and mental disorders: findings from the California Quality of Life Survey. BMC Psychiatr 2009;9:52.
11. Lauver DR, Karon SL, Egan J, et al. Understanding Lesbians' mammography utilization. Wom Health Issues 1999;9:264–74.
12. Case P, Austin SB, Hunter DJ, et al. Sexual orientation, health risk factors and physical functioning in the Nurses' Health Study II. J Women's Health 2004;13:1033–47.
13. Conron KJ, Mimiaga MJ, Landers SJ. A population based study of sexual orientation, identity and gender differences in adult health. Am J Public Health 2010; 100(10):1953–60.
14. Deraz O, Caceres BA, Streed CG, et al. Sexual minority status disparities in Life's Essential 8 and Life's Simple 7 cardiovascular health scores: a French Nationwide population-based study. J Am Heart Assoc 2023;12(11). https://doi.org/10.1161/jaha.122.028429.
15. VanKim NA, Austin SB, Jun HJ, et al. Physical activity and sedentary behaviors among lesbian, bisexual and heterosexual women: findings from the Nurses' Health Study II. J Women's Health 2017;26:1077–85.
16. Blosnich JR, Farmer GW, Lee JGL, et al. Health inequalities among sexual minority adults: evidence from ten U.S. States. Am J Public Health 2014;46(4):337–49.
17. Caceres BA, Brody AA, Halkitis PN, et al. Cardiovascular disease risk in sexual minority women (18-59 years old): findings form the National Health and Nutrition Examination Survey (2001-2012). Wom Health Issues 2018;28(4):333–41.
18. Substance Abuse and Mental Health Services Administration. 2021-2022 lesbian, gay and bisexual behavioral health report. Rockville, MD: Center for Behavioral

Health Statistics and Quality; 2023. https://www.samhsa.gov/data/report/LGB-Behavioral-Health-Report-2021-2022.
19. Fredriksen-Goldsen KI, Emlet CA, Kim HJ, et al. The physical and mental health of lesbian, gay male and bisexual (LGB) older adults: the role of key health indicators and risk and protective factors. Gerontol 2012;53(4):664–75.
20. Fredriksen-Goldsen KI, Kim HJ, Emlet CA, et al. The Aging and Health Report: Resilience and disparities among Lesbian, Gay, Bisexual and Transgender Older Adults. New York. 2011.
21. Mays VM, Cochran SD. Mental health correlates of perceived discrimination among lesbian, gay and bisexual adults in the United States. Am J Public Health 2001;91(11):1869–76.
22. Jen S. Smoking among older sexual minority women: effects of age and sexual orientation. Gerontol 2016;56(Suppl_3):80.
23. Choi SK, Meyer IH. LGBT Aging: a review of research findings, needs and policy implications. Los Angeles: The Williams Institute; 2016.
24. Rowan GA, Frimpong EY, Mengxuan L, et al. Health disparities between older lesbian, gay and bisexual adults and heterosexual adults in the public mental health system. Psychiatr Serv 2022;73(1):39–45.
25. Duncan DT, Zweig S, Hambrick HR, et al. Sexual orientation disparities in prescription opioid misuse among U.S. Adults. Am J Prev Med 2019;56(1):17–26.
26. Schuler MS, Collins RL. Sexual minority substance use disparities: bisexual women at elevated risk relative to other sexual minority groups. Drug Alcohol Depend 2020;206:107755.
27. Lee JH, Garamel KE, Bryant KJ, et al. Discrimination, mental health and substance use disorders among sexual minority populations. LGBT Healt 2016;3(4):258–65.
28. Zivony A, Saguy T. Stereotype deduction about bisexual women. J Sex Res 2018; 55(4–5):666–78.
29. Feinstein BA, Dyar C. Bisexuality, minority stress and health. Curr Sex Health Rep 2017;9(1):42–9.
30. Botswick WB, Dodge B. Introduction to the special section on bisexual health: can you see us now? Arch Sex Behav 2019;481(1):79–87.
31. Friedman MR, Dodge B, Schick V, et al. From bias to bisexual health disparities: attitudes towards bisexual men and women in the United States. LGBT Health 2014;1(4):309–18.
32. Cochran SD, Mays VM, Bowen D, et al. Cancer-related risk indicators among preventative screening behaviors among lesbians and bisexual women. Am J Public Health 2001;91:591–7.
33. Kerker BD, Mostashari F, Thorpe L. Health care access and utilization among women who have sex with women: sexual behavior and identity. J Urban Health 2006;83(5):970–9.
34. Rankow EJ, Tessaro I. Cervical cancer risk and Papanicolaou screening in a sample of lesbian and bisexual women. J Fam Pract 1998;47:139–43.
35. Diamant AL, Wold C, Spritzer K, et al. Health behaviors, health status, and access to and use of health care: a population-based study of lesbian, bisexual and heterosexual women. Arch Fam Med 2000;9:1043–51.
36. Valanis BG. Sexual orientation and health: comparisons in the women's health Initiative sample. Arch Fam Med 2000;9(9):843–53.
37. Meads C, Moore D. Breast cancer in lesbians and bisexual women: systematic review of incidence, prevalence and risk studies. BMC Publ Health 2013;13:1127.
38. Juster RP, McEwen BS, Lupien SJ. Allostatic load biomarkers of chronic stress and impact on health and cognition. Neurosci Biobehav Rev 2010;35(1):2–16.

39. Correro AN, Nielson KA. A review of minority stress as a risk factor for cognitive decline in lesbian, gay, bisexual and transgender (LGBT) elders. J Gay Lesb Ment Health 2020;24(1):2–19.
40. Alzheimer's Association and SAGE. Issue Brief: LGBT and Dementia. 2018. Accessed 13 Aug 2023. https://www.alz.org/media/documents/lgbt-dementia-issues-brief.pdf.
41. Fredriksen-Goldsen KI, Jen S, Bryan AE, et al. Cognitive impairment, Alzheimer's Disease, and other dementias in the lives of lesbian, gay, bisexual and transgender older adults and their caregivers. J Appl Gerontol 2018;37(5):545–69.
42. Hsieh N, Liu H, Wen-Hua L. Elevated risk of cognitive impairment among older sexual minorities: do health conditions, health behaviors and social connections matter? Gerontol 2021;61(3):352–62.
43. Flatt JD, Johnson JK, Karpiak SE, et al. Correlates of subjective cognitive decline in lesbian, gay, bisexual, and transgender older adults. J Alzheim Dis 2018;64(1): 91–102.
44. Nelson CL, Andel R. Does sexual orientation relate to health and well-being? An analysis of adults 50+ years of age. Gerontol 2020;60(7):1282–90.
45. Perales-Puchalt J, Gauthreaux K, Flatt J, et al. Risk of dementia and mild cognitive impairment among older adults in same-sex relationships. Int J Geri Psych 2019;34(6):828–35.
46. Equal Rights Center. Opening Doors: An Investigation of Barriers to Senior Housing for Same-Sex Couples. Washington, D.C. 2014.
47. SAGE. Disrupting Disparities: Solutions for LGBTQ New Yorkers Age 50+. New York, NY. 2021. https://www.sageusa.org/resource-posts/disrupting-disparities-solutions-for-lgbtq-new-yorkers-50/.
48. AARP Research. Dignity 2022: The Experience of LGBTQ Older Adults. Washington, D.C. 2022 https://www.aarp.org/content/dam/aarp/research/surveys_statistics/life-leisure/2022/lgbtq-community-dignity-2022-report.doi.10.26419-2Fres.00549.001.pdf.
49. Kim HJ, Fredriksen-Goldsen KI. Living arrangement and loneliness among lesbian, gay and bisexual older adults. Gerontol 2016;56(3):548–58.
50. SAGE. National Coming Out Day: Some LGBTQ+ seniors fearing discrimination go back 'into the closet'. 2011. Accessed 23 Aug 2023. https://www.sageusa.org/news-posts/national-coming-out-day-some-lgbtq-seniors-fearing-discrimination-go-back-into-the-closet/.

Gender-Affirming Care for Older Transgender and Gender Diverse Adults

Asa E. Radix, MD, PhD, MPH[a,b,c,*], Loren Schechter, MD[d], Alexander B. Harris, MPH, CPH[a], Zil Goldstein, MSN, RN, FNP[a,e]

KEYWORDS

- Transgender • Gender-affirming care • Aging • Geriatric • Nonbinary

KEY POINTS

- Transgender older adults have been described as both "underserved and understudied."
- For transgender people, aging comes with a unique set of challenges and experiences, including health care disparities, mental health concerns, and social isolation.
- It is crucial for clinicians to understand and address the specific needs of aging transgender individuals by providing evidence-based quality health care, including preventive screenings, offering mental health support, and advocating for legal protections.

INTRODUCTION

In the United States, approximately 1.6 million adults identify as transgender, meaning they have a gender identity that does not align with the sex assigned to them at birth.[1] Although there are limited data about older transgender and gender diverse people, the Williams Institute estimates that 0.3% of Americans aged 65 and older, or almost 172,000 individuals, identify as transgender.[1]

Transgender older adults have been described as both "underserved and understudied."[2] The landmark Institute of Medicine (IOM) Report on The Health of Lesbian, Gay, Bisexual, and Transgender People noted that very little was known about transgender aging, as much of the literature and research about aging in sexual and gender minority (SGM) populations often does not include transgender and gender diverse (TGD) people.[3] Similarly, guidelines that address clinical care of transgender people

[a] Callen-Lorde Community Health Center, 356 West 18th Street, New York, NY 10011, USA; [b] Department of Epidemiology, Mailman School of Public Health, 722 West 168th Street, New York, NY 10032, USA; [c] Department of Medicine, NYU Grossman School of Medicine, NY, USA; [d] Rush University Medical Center, Rush University, 1725 West Harrison Street, Suite 758, Chicago, IL 60612, USA; [e] CUNY School of Public Health and Health Policy, 55 West 125TH Street, New York, NY 10027, USA
* Corresponding author.
E-mail address: aradix@callen-lorde.org

Clin Geriatr Med 40 (2024) 261–271
https://doi.org/10.1016/j.cger.2023.12.002
0749-0690/24/

do not include specific guidance for the care of transgender people as they age.[4] Over the last decade since the IOM report was published, there has been a steady increase in the number of publications related to transgender health. However, most literature has focused on topics related to mental health and substance use as well as sexual and reproductive health. Far fewer studies have investigated general health topics, including issues related to aging for TGD people.[5] As the number of transgender persons age, providers need to be equipped to understand their unique circumstances and medical needs.

HISTORICAL PERSPECTIVES

Over the last few decades, increased visibility and awareness of transgender people has resulted in greater acceptance in society and improved civil rights protections, yet much work remains. Transgender individuals who are greater than 65 years of age faced a societal landscape that was even more challenging than today. In one study of LGBT older adults (Care and Aging with Pride), over 90% of older transgender individuals had been victimized at least once (including verbal assault, physical threats, and physical assault), and 78% had experienced 3 or more incidents.[6] For many trans elders, access to gender-affirming care was extremely limited, in part due to a lack of knowledgeable medical providers who offered transition-related medical care. Historically, most third-party payers, both public and private, deemed gender-affirming hormones and surgeries "cosmetic," and excluded coverage. In 2014, that the Department of Health and Human Services lifted the Medicare exclusion on gender-affirming care and began reimbursement for services that were considered medically necessary services on a case-by-case basis.[7,8] Subsequently, there was a significant increase in Medicare-eligible individuals accessing care, including gender-affirming surgeries.[9] Increased uptake of gender-affirming care similarly occurred after commercial insurance and state Medicaid plans started to cover the costs of gender-affirming care as a result of state-level anti-discrimination bills. The nondiscrimination clause of the 2010 Patient Protection and Affordable Care Act gave grounds to legally challenge remaining insurance restrictions, creating an insurance coverage pathway for thousands of transgender people to pay for gender-affirming care.[7,10,11]

Clinicians caring for older transgender adults need to understand the many ways that past experiences of discrimination, including in health care settings, and the lack of culturally competent and appropriate care have negatively impacted their physical and mental health as well as their trust in the medical systems.

CLINICAL CARE CONSIDERATIONS FOR AGING TRANSGENDER INDIVIDUALS

Several studies examining determinates of health and care outcomes among older transgender adults have found an elevated burden of chronic disease and poor mental health in this population. In the Care and Aging with Pride study of older LGBT adults, transgender individuals faced high rates of disability (62%), depression (48%), and financial barriers to care (22%) and compared with LGB adults, were more likely to experience poverty and social isolation.[6] A study of Medicare beneficiaries found that 88.2% of transgender Medicare beneficiaries had multiple chronic conditions, compared with 72.4% of their cisgender counterparts. Transgender members were noted to have higher rates of certain mood disorders (anxiety, depression, and post-traumatic stress disorder [PTSD]), human immunodeficiency virus(HIV), asthma, chronic obstructive pulmonary disease, stroke, and substance use.[12] Many aging transgender persons rely on social and medical services to manage these medical conditions. Despite this, multiple studies have shown that medical providers and trainees often lack the skills and knowledge to appropriately care for transgender individuals longitudinally, including provision of gender-affirming care, management of chronic conditions, and oversight of their general health needs such as cancer screening.[13–18]

GENERAL APPROACH TO CARE

The high rates of trauma and PTSD in this population necessitate taking a trauma-informed approach to care. Trauma and PTSD influence HIV risk and pre-exposure prophylaxis uptake and likely have effects on other aspects of health.[19] Using the basics of trauma-informed care and maintaining transparency about care decisions and shared decision-making techniques will enhance both the relationship with the older transgender patient and help them access care. Engaging with patients, recognizing their past trauma and acting with empathy, trustworthiness, offering choices with health decisions, and empowering the patient to advocate for their health will open more possibilities when working with traumatized patients. Something as simple as explaining the lab tests being done in every patient visit and why they are important can help patients build trust in their provider and become more empowered in their health. Offering choices such as delivery method for hormone therapy, choice of blood pressure medication, or best treatment for diabetes allows the patient to take ownership of their health instead of being a passive recipient of care. These steps allow traumatized patients to feel as though they have some level of control of their health care and will help them to begin to explore other health possibilities.

GENDER-AFFIRMING INTERVENTIONS FOR AGING TRANSGENDER PEOPLE

Many transgender individuals seek out gender-affirming hormone therapy or surgical interventions to align their secondary sex characteristics and/or anatomy with their affirmed gender.[4] In recent years, an increasing number of older transgender individuals have accessed gender-affirming interventions for the first time. Early evidence shows that quality of life measures (QoL) are positively impacted for this age group, and that older transgender individuals demonstrate higher QoL compared to younger transgender individuals who are initiating this care.[20]

Individuals assigned female at birth who identify as nonbinary, male, or on the transmasculine spectrum may request testosterone therapy. There are many formulations of testosterone, including injectable (either intramuscular or subcutaneous) testosterone cypionate or enanthate, intramuscular testosterone undecanoate, and testosterone gel, among others (**Table 1**). The regimens are thought to be equivalent, and the decision about the mode of administration made after consideration of patient preference, cost, and insurance coverage. Testosterone treatment has several effects including the development of facial hair and body hair, deepening of the voice, a redistribution of facial and body fat, an increase in muscle mass, clitoral enlargement, and occasionally androgenetic hair loss.[4]

Individuals assigned male at birth who identify as nonbinary, female, or on the trans-feminine spectrum may request estrogen preparations, for example, estradiol tablets, estradiol cypionate or estradiol valerate injection, or transdermal estradiol (patch).[4] In addition, if the patient has testes, an androgen blocker is usually indicated to suppress serum testosterone levels to less than 50 ng/dL (see **Table 1**). In the United States, spironolactone, in doses up to 300 mg daily, is the most frequently androgen blocker. Other androgen blockers include 5 alpha reductase inhibitors, such as finasteride or dutasteride, or gonadotropin-releasing hormone agonists such as leuprolide.[4,21] General effects of feminizing hormone therapy include breast development, a redistribution of facial and

Table 1
Gender-affirming hormone therapy

Regimens for Transmasculine Individuals		
Testosterone Therapy	Testosterone Cypionate/ Enanthate	50–100 mg every week SC or 100–200 mg every 2 wk IM
	Testosterone Undecanoate	750 mg IM every 10 wk
	Testosterone Gel	50–100 mg/day
Regimens for Transfeminine Individuals		
Estrogen Therapy	Estradiol Tablets	2.0–6.0 mg/day PO
	Estradiol Transdermal Patch	0.025–0.2 mg/day
	Estradiol Valerate/Cypionate	5–30 mg IM every 2 wk 2–10 IM every week
Androgen Blockers[a]	Spironolactone	100–300 mg/day PO
	Finasteride	1–5 mg/day PO
	Leuprolide	3.75–7.50 mg SQ/IM monthly

Abbreviations: IM, intramuscular; PO, oral; SC, subcutaneous.
[a] For individuals with gonads.
Adapted from: Coleman at al. IJTH, 2022 and UCSF Primary Care Protocols.[4,21]

body fat, reduction of muscle mass, softening of the skin, possible reversal of androgenetic hair loss, erectile dysfunction, and reduced sperm count.[4]

There are currently no data on efficacy of gender-affirming hormones in older age groups compared to younger individuals, and most of the dose modifications in older individuals are to mitigate adverse effects, for example, transdermal estradiol as the preferred estrogen to reduce venous thromboembolism, or lower doses of spironolactone to avoid hypotension. Additionally, there are no recommendations to reduce or stop hormones as patients age unless there are medical indications to do so. Patients may choose to stop hormone regimens due to non-medical reasons, for example, cost or personal preference. Clinicians should caution patients that stopping hormones after undergoing gonadectomy can accelerate bone loss, and close monitoring will be needed. The choice of regimen is made after consideration of patient preference, cost, and insurance coverage. For individuals aged 45 or older, the preferred estrogen is transdermal estradiol, since this is associated with a lower risk of venous thromboembolism compared to other estrogen formulations. Older adults, especially those with co-occurring medical conditions, such as chronic kidney disease, may not tolerate the high doses of spironolactone used for androgen suppression. Hyperkalemia, although an uncommon occurrence, may be a greater risk to individuals who are taking other medications that can also result in high serum potassium, such as angiotensin-converting enzyme inhibitors (ACE inhibitors). Apart from the recommendation about use of transdermal estradiol, The World Professional Association of Transgender Health (WPATH) Standards of Care does not have any preferred hormone or dosing regimens for older transgender adults.

When counseling patients about the risks and benefits of gender-affirming hormone therapy, patients should be informed about the increased risk of venous thromboembolism and cardiovascular disease with estrogen, especially in older adults.[22] Patients should be counseled on strategies to reduce risk, such as smoking cessation and optimization of lipid control with statins and healthy lifestyle interventions.

Monitoring hormone therapy usually occurs at least every 3 months in the first year after initiation and at least once or twice each year thereafter.[4] The medical provider should document any reported physical or mood changes or adverse effects related to the hormone regimen. Providers should enquire about symptoms, such as dizziness or orthostasis, that may occur in older individuals receiving spironolactone. Laboratory monitoring should include serum estradiol and testosterone levels for individuals using estrogens and androgen blockers, and a serum testosterone level and hematocrit for individuals on testosterone treatment. If spironolactone is used, then monitoring of renal function and serum potassium is indicated. The timing of laboratory tests is important, with a mid-cycle or trough level recommended for injectable hormones.[4]

Some individuals may want to undergo gender-affirming surgeries to align their physical characteristics with their gender identity. Gender-affirming surgeries for transfeminine individuals are numerous and may include breast augmentation, body contouring, facial surgery, vocal cord surgery, vaginoplasty (creation of a vagina usually with penile/scrotal skin, peritoneum, or intestinal flaps and grafts), orchiectomy, vulvoplasty (creation of clitorovulvar structures without the construction of a vaginal canal), and body contouring, in addition to procedures, such as hair removal or hair grafting. Procedures for transmasculine individuals may include bilateral mastectomy (also called top surgery), facial surgery, vocal cord surgery, phalloplasty, metoidioplasty (with or without urethral lengthening and/or placement of penile and testicular prostheses), scrotoplasty, hysterectomy, vaginectomy, and body contouring (**Table 2**). Although there is limited information about the number of older transgender adults who undertake these procedures, Medicare reveals that the number of patients accessing gender-affirming surgeries increased 3-fold between the years 2012 to 2013 and 2014.[9] Using 2016 to 2020 data from the Nationwide Ambulatory Surgery Sample and the National Inpatient Sample, it is estimated that 4406 transgender individuals in the United States aged over 50 years accessed gender-affirming surgeries, equivalent to 0.5% of the 48,019 individuals undergoing gender-affirming procedures in that time frame.[23] Of older adults, 1336 (30.3%) accessed breast/chest surgeries (breast augmentation or mastectomy), 2414 (54.8%) accessed genital surgeries, and 858 (19%) other procedures. It is noteworthy that 126 individuals over the age of 70 years undertook genital surgeries.[23]

The primary care provider plays an important role in the care of patients who are planning for or who have undergone gender-affirming surgeries. In the pre-operative period, this includes referrals for hair removal before genital surgery, optimization of medical conditions, and pre-operative risk assessment. Additionally, the primary care provider may help prepare people for surgery by reviewing their post-surgical care plan (including post-operative support, activity restrictions, time off work, financial considerations, etc…). After surgery, the provider can assist patients with ongoing follow-up care, identification of and referrals for surgery-related complications, and preventive care screening (described below). Most complications following gender-affirming surgery are self-limited and treated on an outpatient basis. The most common early complications are wound disruptions, typically treated with local wound care. As with any surgical procedure, other complications include infection (skin, soft tissue, urinary, and respiratory), usually treated with oral antibiotics, tissue loss (which may require secondary and/or revision procedures), bleeding/hematoma, and venous thromboembolism. Each procedure carries surgery-specific risks. For example, phalloplasty may be associated with urethral stricture/fistula or flap failure resulting in loss of the reconstructed phallus.[24] Risks of vaginoplasty include vaginal stenosis, urinary stream abnormalities (ie, spraying, meatal stenosis), fistula (rectovaginal or urethrovaginal), granulation tissue (generally amenable to treatment with silver nitrate), tissue loss (graft loss, clitoral necrosis), and vaginal prolapse..[25] The primary care provider should have a low threshold for referring patients back to their primary surgeon or for urgent/emergent evaluation if serious postoperative complications occur, especially within the first month.

Table 2
Descriptions of common gender-affirming surgeries

Surgical Procedure	Description
Breast Augmentation	Similar to breast augmentation procedures in cisgender women. Often uses subpectoral placement of implants
Chondrolaryngoplasty	Thyroid cartilage (Adam's apple) reduction
Facial Feminization Surgery	Includes an array of surgeries such as mandibular angle reduction, forehead contouring, rhinoplasty, blepharoplasty, cheek, or lip augmentation
Metoidioplasty	Surgery to lengthen the hormonally enlarged clitoris by release of clitoral attachments
Phalloplasty	Construction of a penis using tissue from the forearm (radial forearm free flap), thigh (anterior lateral thigh), upper back (musculocutaneous latissimus dorsi flap), or lower abdomen (pedicled abdominal flap). Penile prostheses, for example, malleable rods or inflatable devices, are used to achieve erectile function
Scrotoplasty	Construction of a scrotum using the labia majora. Testicular implants may be inserted
Top Surgery/Chest Masculinization	Bilateral mastectomy usually with relocation of the nipple-areola complex
Urethroplasty	Lengthening of the urethra within the shaft of the new penis, using skin, buccal, or vaginal grafts that allows the individual to void while standing
Vaginectomy	Surgery to remove the vagina epithelium with obliteration of the vaginal canal. This surgery can only be done after a hysterectomy.
Vaginoplasty	Construction of a vagina usually using penile skin or intestinal grafts or peritoneal flap
Vocal cord surgery	Surgery to modify the vocal cords to elevate or lower pitch
Vulvoplasty	Construction of the female external genitalia only without a vaginal canal. Also called "zero depth" vaginoplasty

There are no specific recommendations for cancer screening in individuals who have had genital gender-affirming surgeries. Squamous cell carcinoma has been reported in women who have had penile-inversion vaginoplasty.[26] In those who had vaginoplasty using intestinal grafts, there is a remote possibility of neovaginal adenocarcinoma.[27] Providers should be aware of symptoms, such as bleeding, pain, excess vaginal discharge, that may indicate a need for further evaluation. Vaginal inspection can be performed using a small speculum and is recommended as part of routine follow-up care, although the frequency of examination has not been determined.

SEXUAL HEALTH

Clinicians are often reluctant to discuss sexual health with older patients despite knowing that sexual health is an important metric of quality of life.[28] Medical providers may face even more challenges initiating discussions with aging transgender patients due to their own discomfort and limited knowledge about the impact of gender-affirming interventions on sexual function. It is important for medical providers to normalize discussions about sexual health and to elicit sexual health concerns with transgender patients. Providers need to be aware of the higher rates of sexual trauma, violence, and PTSD in this population and ensure to use best practices of trauma-informed care. Transgender individuals who use estrogen and androgen blockers may experience erectile dysfunction and low libido. Medical providers may need to adjust reduce the androgen-blocker dose to alleviate these symptoms. Adding low-dose transdermal testosterone, to achieve a serum testosterone level 25 to 100 ng/dL, may reduce symptoms for those who have had gonadectomy. Over 80% of individuals who undergo vaginoplasty are able to achieve orgasm, and the majority report general sexual satisfaction.[29] Postoperative complications, such as vaginal stenosis, can cause pain with sexual activity. Individuals who use testosterone treatment usually experience increased libido; however, testosterone is also associated with pelvic pain and vaginal dryness resulting in discomfort during sexual activity.[30] Vaginal estrogen and pelvic physical therapy may be options to reduce testosterone-related pain.

GENDER-AFFIRMING CARE AT THE END OF LIFE AND PALLIATIVE CARE

The number of transgender individuals in the United States has steadily increased over time, reflecting greater societal acceptance and improved access to gender-affirming care. As these individuals age, there is a need for medical providers and health systems to consider their unique concerns, including provision of culturally appropriate end-of-life care.

Aging transgender individuals have particular concerns related to end of life including not being able to care for themselves and being directed into long-term

Table 3
Resources for aging transgender persons

FORGE - Transgender Aging Network	FORGE hosts a support and networking e-mail ElderTG: an email list for transgender persons age 50+	https://forge-forward.org/resource/Transgender-Aging-network/
GLMA– Health Professionals Advancing LGBTQ + Equality	A professional network committed to ensuring health equity for lesbian, gay, bisexual, transgender, and queer (LGBTQ+) communities	GLMA Provider Directory https://www.glma.org/find_a_provider.php
Lambda Legal	US civil rights organization that focuses on LGBT communities	FAQ For Transgender and Gender-Nonconforming Older Adults https://legacy.lambdalegal.org/know-your-rights/article/trans-seniors-faq
SAGE (Services and Advocacy for LGBTQ + Elders)	National advocacy and services organization for LGBTQ + elders	Website: https://www.sageusa.org/SAGE Hotline: 877–360-LGBT(5428)
Transgender Care Listings	A list of affirming medical and mental health services	http://transcaresite.org/
World Professional Association for Transgender Health (WPATH)	An interdisciplinary professional and educational organization devoted to transgender health. WPATH hosts a provider directory	https://www.wpath.org/provider/search

care facilities. In these settings, people worry about discrimination, being disrespected on the basis of their gender identity, and/or being unable to express their identity as they age. Another fear is lack of access to gender-affirming care and discontinuation of hormone medications.[31–34] Other discriminatory actions included mistreatment of the patient's spouse or partner, including being denied access to the patient when they were in intensive care or emergency department settings.[35]

If patients need to enter nursing homes or other institutions, they should be reassured regarding their right to continuation of medically necessary gender-affirming care and protections are in place against discrimination on the basis of gender identity (**Table 3** resources). The WPATH Standards of Care 8 reaffirms the right of transgender individuals in institutional settings to receive gender-affirming hormone therapy and surgical interventions, and to receive appropriate monitoring of gender-related care. These recommendations underscore the importance of institutions addressing transgender people by their chosen names and pronouns at all times.

SUMMARY

For transgender people, aging comes with a unique set of challenges and experiences, including health care disparities, mental health concerns, and social isolation. It is crucial for clinicians to understand and address the specific needs of aging transgender individuals by providing evidence-based quality health care, including preventive screenings, offering mental health support, and advocating for legal protections. In doing so, they can create a more inclusive and equitable society where transgender adults can age with dignity and pride.

CLINICS CARE POINTS

Clinicians should follow established best practices to ensure that older transgender patients receive high-quality and culturally appropriate health care. These include.

- Use inclusive language: Patients should be addressed using their chosen name and pronoun. These should be clearly documented in their medical records to avoid harm to the patient through misgendering (using incorrect pronouns). One of the key factors that has been shown to improve utilization of preventive care services is having an affirming primary care provider.[36]
- Stay informed about advances in transgender medicine though continuing education. New research findings have the potential to improve current medical practice. Clinicians can stay abreast of new recommendations by participating in transgender health courses, for example, those offered by professional societies including WPATH.[37]
- Maintain an up-to-date anatomic inventory and document both the gender identity and the sex assigned at birth in medical records. This will allow clinicians to provide appropriate anatomy-based screening, for example, to identify a transgender man who has a cervix who requires cervical cancer screening.
- Assess mental health concerns and make appropriate referrals to affirming mental health services. Older transgender individuals have higher rates of depression, anxiety, and post-traumatic stress disorder. Providers should endeavor to screen for these conditions.
- Ask about experiences with health care, including past discrimination. Understanding past experiences will provide insight into potential barriers to care and allow opportunities to provide additional support. For example, a patient who has experienced problems picking up prescriptions due to a mismatch between their chosen name and legal name can be provided with resources for low-cost or free legal name change services.

- **Social Support and Resilience:** Social support, including friends, chosen families, and LGBTQ + community organizations, plays a crucial role in transgender individuals' ability to thrive in later life. Finding a supportive network can mitigate the effects of discrimination and isolation. Clinicians can assist by providing resources to support groups, either in person or online, and referrals to affirming providers (see resources **Table 3**)
- **Address End of Life care and Advance Care Planning:** Older transgender persons may not have adequate resources set aside for their end of life, partly due to lifelong economic marginalization. They may also have neglected to designate a durable power of attorney for health care decisions. Clinicians should discuss EOL planning and provide patients with resources from organizations that serve older LGBT people, such as . Services and Advocacy for LGBTQ + Elders (SAGE) (see **Table 3**).[38]
- Reassure patients of their right to have medically necessary gender-affirming care continued in long-term care facilities.

DISCLOSURE

The authors have no financial disclosures to declare.

FUNDING

Dr Radix is supported by the National Institute of Mental Health under award number R25MH087217.

REFERENCES

1. Herman JL, Flores, A.R., O'Neill, K.K. How Many Adults and Youth Identify as Transgender in the United States? 2022. https://williamsinstitute.law.ucla.edu/wp-content/uploads/Trans-Pop-Update-Jun-2022.pdf.
2. Persson DI. Unique challenges of transgender aging: implications from the literature. J Gerontol Soc Work 2009;52(6):633–46. https://doi.org/10.1080/01634370802609056.
3. Institute of Medicine (US) Committee on Lesbian. Gay, Bisexual, and Transgender Health Issues and Research Gaps and Opportunities. *The health of lesbian, gay,. and transgender people building a foundation for better understanding.* Washington, DC: National Academies Press; 2011. p. xviii, 347.
4. Coleman E, Radix AE, Bouman WP, et al. Standards of care for the health of transgender and gender diverse people, version 8. International Journal of Transgender Health 2022;23(sup1):S1–259.
5. Reisner SL, Deutsch MB, Bhasin S, et al. Advancing methods for US transgender health research. Curr Opin Endocrinol Diabetes Obes 2016;23(2):198–207.
6. Fredriksen-Goldsen KI, Kim H, Emlet CA, et al. The aging and health report: Disparities and resilience among lesbian, gay, bisexual, and transgender older adults. 2011. http://caringandaging.org/wordpress/wp-content/uploads/2012/10/Full-report10-25-12.pdf.
7. Baker KE. The future of transgender coverage. N Engl J Med 2017;376(19):1801–4.
8. Sussan LA, Hegy, S. A., Tobias, C. B.,. National Coverage Determination - 140.3, Transsexual Surgery. In: Services. USDoHaH, editor. 2014.
9. Canner JK, Harfouch O, Kodadek LM, et al. Temporal trends in gender-affirming surgery among transgender patients in the United States. JAMA surgery 2018;153(7):609–16.

10. Nondiscrimination in health programs and activities. Final rule. Fed Regist 2016; 81(96):31375–473.
11. Wiegmann AL, Young EI, Baker KE, et al. The affordable care Act and its impact on plastic and gender-affirmation surgery. Plast Reconstr Surg 2021;147(1): 135e–53e.
12. Dragon CN, Guerino P, Ewald E, et al. Transgender Medicare beneficiaries and chronic conditions: exploring fee-for-service claims data. LGBT Health 2017; 4(6):404–11. https://doi.org/10.1089/lgbt.2016.0208.
13. Unger CA. Care of the transgender patient: a survey of gynecologists' current knowledge and practice. J Womens Health (Larchmt) 2015;24(2):114–8. https://doi.org/10.1089/jwh.2014.4918.
14. Chisolm-Straker M, Willging C, Daul AD, et al. Transgender and gender-nonconforming patients in the emergency department: what physicians know, think, and do. Ann Emerg Med 2018;71(2):183–8.e1. https://doi.org/10.1016/j.annemergmed.2017.09.042.
15. Sherman ADF, McDowell A, Clark KD, et al. Transgender and gender diverse health education for future nurses: students' knowledge and attitudes. Nurse Educ Today 2021;97:104690.
16. Vasudevan A, García AD, Hart BG, et al. Health professions students' knowledge, skills, and attitudes toward transgender healthcare. J Community Health 2022; 47(6):981–9.
17. Christopherson L, McLaren K, Schramm L, et al. Assessment of knowledge, comfort, and skills working with transgender clients of saskatchewan family physicians, family medicine residents, and nurse practitioners. Transgend Health 2022;7(5):468–72.
18. Carroll EF, Woodard GA, St Amand CM, et al. Breast cancer screening recommendations for transgender and gender diverse patients: a knowledge and familiarity assessment of primary care practitioners. J Community Health 2023;48(5): 889–97.
19. Storholm ED, Huang W, Ogunbajo A, et al. Gender-based violence and post-traumatic stress disorder symptoms predict HIV PrEP uptake and persistence failure among transgender and non-binary persons participating in a PrEP demonstration project in southern California. AIDS Behav 2023;27(2):745–59.
20. Cai X, Hughto JMW, Reisner SL, et al. Benefit of gender-affirming medical treatment for transgender elders: later-life alignment of mind and body. LGBT Health 2019;6(1):34–9.
21. Center of Excellence for Transgender Health DoFaCM, University of California San Francisco,. Deutsch M, ed. Guidelines for the Primary and Gender-Affirming Care of Transgender and Gender Nonbinary People. 2nd ed. University of California San Francisco; 2016. Updated June 2016. Accessed 12/20/2018. www.transhealth.ucsf.edu/.
22. Spyridoula M, Naykky SO, Rene R-G, et al. Sex steroids and cardiovascular outcomes in transgender individuals: a systematic review and meta-analysis. J Clin Endocrinol Metabol 2017;9(102):3914–23.
23. Wright JD, Chen L, Suzuki Y, et al. National estimates of gender-affirming surgery in the US. JAMA Netw Open 2023;6(8):e2330348.
24. Heston AL, Esmonde NO, Dugi DD 3rd, et al. Phalloplasty: techniques and outcomes. Transl Androl Urol 2019;8(3):254–65.
25. Hontscharuk R, Alba B, Hamidian Jahromi A, et al. Penile inversion vaginoplasty outcomes: complications and satisfaction. Andrology 2021;9(6):1732–43.

26. Fierz R, Ghisu GP, Fink D. Squamous carcinoma of the neovagina after male-to-female reconstruction surgery: a case report and review of the literature. Case Rep Obstet Gynecol 2019;2019:4820396.
27. Yamada K, Shida D, Kato T, et al. Adenocarcinoma arising in sigmoid colon neovagina 53 years after construction. World J Surg Oncol 2018;16(1):88.
28. Malta S, Hocking J, Lyne J, et al. Do you talk to your older patients about sexual health? Health practitioners' knowledge of, and attitudes towards, management of sexual health among older Australians. Aust J Gen Pract 2018;47(11):807–11.
29. Morrison SD, Claes K, Morris MP, et al. Principles and outcomes of gender-affirming vaginoplasty. Nat Rev Urol 2023;20(5):308–22.
30. Tordoff DM, Lunn MR, Chen B, et al. Testosterone use and sexual function among transgender men and gender diverse people assigned female at birth. Am J Obstet Gynecol 2023. https://doi.org/10.1016/j.ajog.2023.08.035.
31. Catlett L, Acquaviva KD, Campbell L, et al. End-of-Life care for transgender older adults. Glob Qual Nurs Res Jan-2023;10. https://doi.org/10.1177/23333936231161128. 23333936231161128.
32. Witten TM. End of life, chronic illness, and trans-identities. J Soc Work End Life Palliat Care 2014;10(1):34–58.
33. Henry RS, Perrin PB, Coston BM, et al. Transgender and gender non-conforming adult preparedness for aging: concerns for aging, and familiarity with and engagement in planning behaviors. Int J Transgend Health 2020;21(1):58–69.
34. Witten TM. It's not all darkness: robustness, resilience, and successful transgender aging. *LGBT health.* Mar 2014;1(1):24–33.
35. Stein GL, Berkman C, O'Mahony S, et al. Experiences of lesbian, Gay, bisexual, and transgender patients and families in hospice and palliative care: perspectives of the palliative care team. J Palliat Med 2020;23(6):817–24.
36. McKay T, Tran NM, Barbee H, et al. Association of affirming care with chronic disease and preventive care outcomes among lesbian, Gay, bisexual, transgender, and queer older adults. Am J Prev Med 2023;64(3):305–14. https://doi.org/10.1016/j.amepre.2022.09.025.
37. World Professional Association of Transgender Health. https://www.wpath.org/
38. SAGE. Advocacy and Services for LGBTQ+ Elders. https://www.sageusa.org/.

Primary Care and Health Care of Transgender and Gender-Diverse Older Adults

Wendy J. Chen, MD[a,b,*], Asa E. Radix, MD, PhD, MPH[c,d]

KEYWORDS

• Transgender • Gender diverse • Primary care • Screening

KEY POINTS

- It is essential to ensure that care is provided in a safe, affirming, trauma-informed, and welcoming space.
- Clinicians should develop the knowledge and skills to provide clinically and culturally appropriate care to older TGD adults.
- Clinicians should maintain an up-to-date anatomic inventory and discuss age-appropriate health screening for each organ present in a patient-centered manner.
- Older TGD adults receiving gender-affirming hormone therapy require additional monitoring of serum hormone levels and other biomarkers impacted by these regimens, for example, hematocrit or potassium levels.
- Clinicians should prioritize discussions about advance care planning with TGD patients.

BACKGROUND

The outdated term "gender identity disorder (GID)" was used in Diagnostic and Statistical Manual of Mental Disorders (DSM) IV (1994) and DSM IV text revision (TR) (2000). Importantly, this term is no longer used, being replaced by gender dysphoria in the DSM 5 (2013) and remaining the current terminology within the DSM 5-TR (2022). The ICD-11 (2022) recently adopted the term "gender incongruence" to replace transsexualism and GID and relocated the diagnosis from the chapter on mental disorders to the chapter on sexual health. These changes represent significant shifts in perspective, moving away from the view that gender diversity is a mental health disorder, and

[a] Department of Medicine, Loyola University Medicine Center, Chicago, IL, USA; [b] Internal Medicine, ACP AGS WPATH USPATH; [c] Department of Medicine, Callen-Lorde Community Health Center, 356 West 18th Street, New York, NY 10011, USA; [d] Department of Epidemiology, Columbia University Mailman School of Public Health, 722 West 168th Street, New York, NY 10032, USA

* Corresponding author. Division of Hospital Medicine, Loyola University Medical Center, 2160 South 1st Avenue, Maywood, IL 60153.
E-mail address: Dr.wjchen@gmail.com

Clin Geriatr Med 40 (2024) 273–283
https://doi.org/10.1016/j.cger.2023.12.003

thereby reducing stigma associated with this condition. Medically, terminology is ever evolving. When talking to patients or documenting in medical records, it is important to use language that is not dehumanizing or offensive. This can be done by staying abreast of culturally appropriate terms and to take the lead from patients by mirroring language that they use. Key examples include using "sex assigned at birth" instead of "natal sex," and "gender-affirming surgeries" instead of "sex reassignment." Clinicians should also document the patient's affirmed gender consistently using self-described terms, such as Two-spirit, trans man, trans women, etc. to ensure respectful and inclusive care.[1–4]

Environment

Older TGD adults often avoid health care services for a myriad of reasons, including fear of being misgendered or deadnamed (ie, using a previous or legal name instead of chosen name), exposure to inappropriate or transphobic comments, and encounters with medical personnel who are dismissive of their concerns and complaints, coupled with a deficiency in culturally appropriate and competent care.[3,5–8] These negative experiences have been shown to result in delays in both preventive and urgent care.[3,5–7] Creating an environment that is safe and welcoming for all TGD older adults is crucial in establishing positive patient-provider relationships. This experience begins with the patient's first contact, whether that be an appointment reminder or during the patient's initial intake and waiting room experience.

To foster an inclusive environment, physical health care spaces should have lesbian, gay, bisexual, transgender, and questioning (LGBTQ)+-friendly reading material and informational posters. Intake forms should include options for all gender identities, including "other" to allow for patient-defined terminology, in addition to sex assigned at birth, chosen name as well as (legal) name on insurance, and pronouns used.

Additionally, it is beneficial to institute TGD-inclusive procedures for the health care team to ensure affirming care. For instance, having a designated area in the chart and on paperwork used to call patients from the waiting room that distinctly states the patient's used name and pronouns is vital in making TGD patients feel secure and accepted. If a mistake occurs, it is crucial to correct it promptly and apologize. These systems changes not only reinforce a sense of safety and acceptance for TGD individuals but also foster an environment of respect, dignity, and equitable care for all patients.

Beyond inclusive physical environments and in-take procedures, preparation requires education for all staff on both cultural humility and cultural competency care. Clinically, affirming care for TGD has important implications in health care outcomes. For further information on affirming care, please refer to chapter 1.

Transgender Identity and the Comprehensive Geriatric Assessment

As with all geriatric persons, a comprehensive geriatric assessment (CGA) should be utilized to provide high-quality evidence-based health care. The CGA is especially important in TGD patients as they are at a higher risk to experience health care disparities and worse outcomes in each of the CGA domains, even when compared to other minority groups.[3,5,7,9] The authors will highlight some of the trans-specific geriatric needs as a part of the Trans-specific Geriatric Health Assessment (TGHA).

TGD care requires that clinicians understand each individual's unique experiences, particularly for older adults who are navigating their emotions and identities, possibly with conflicting feelings and thoughts. These individuals, under varying societal and familial pressures, may exhibit fluctuating preferences regarding pronouns, names, and transition desires, requiring heightened patience and understanding from health care providers.[3,5–7]

Many older adults may not have previously considered the nuances of gender identity, expression, sexual attraction, or biological sex. Numerous resources are available to aid these discussions (see the "Resources" section) (**Box 1**).

Primary care physicians (PCPs) may need to provide gender documentation for patients, including referral letters and assistance with navigating insurance for gender-affirming interventions. The World Professional Association of Transgender Health (WPATH) Standards of Care 8, which is an international clinical practice guideline, states that the care of TGD patients can be provided by a wide range of health care professionals, including PCPs, who develop the necessary knowledge and skills, and engage in ongoing learning. Providers should be able to adequately assess TGD patients, including to differentiate between mental health issues and gender incongruence or diversity, and be knowledgeable about gender-affirming medical interventions. Otherwise, providers can align with specialists in TGD care to provide this care in a multidisciplinary approach.[4] This comprehensive approach ensures a respectful and responsive health care environment, accommodating the diverse needs of TGD individuals.

Care of older TGD patients includes routine geriatric care, with recommended CGA at initiation of care and annual visits, inclusive of the 4 M's (mobility, mentation, medications, and what matters) of Age Friendly Health Care Systems.[10] For mentation, cognitive assessment can include mini-cog and Montreal Cognitive Assessment. For mobility, instruments like the timed up and go can be used, in addition to noting functional history with activities of daily living (ADLs) and instrumental IADLs and use of assistive device. The CGA should include vision and hearing screenings for any issues, as these can significantly impact daily function and independence. A TGHA should include the ability to dose and give GAHT if applicable.[11] Sleep and nutrition have important impacts on health and mental wellbeing, which make them important to evaluate as well. When collecting medical and sexual histories, understanding a TGD individual's unique experiences and goals is vital, including inquiries about past, current, and potential future gender-affirming medical interventions. It is crucial to acknowledge that some older adults may have resorted to hormones attained outside of medical settings, as well as "herbal hormones," like black cohosh, ashwagandha, or red clover, which can present significant health risks such as liver or kidney injury.[11–13]

Social History

Providers should assess for safety and the presence of a social support system and if the patient lives in a trans-affirming environment as part of TGHA.[4,7,9] TGD older adults often face rejection or limited acceptance from their biological families, leading many

Box 1
Resources

World Professional Association for Transgender Health (WPATH) - www.wpath.org/

Fenway Health, The National LGBTQIA + Health Education Center, the LGBTQIA + Aging Project - https://fenwayhealth.org/

The National LGBTQIA + Health Education Center – https://www.lgbtqiahealtheducation.org/

Endocrine Treatment of Gender-Dysphoric/Gender-Incongruent Persons: An Endocrine Society Clinical Practice Guideline - https://doi.org/10.1210/jc.2017-01658

ARUP Laboratories, Monitoring of Gender-Affirming Hormone Therapy Testing Algorithm https://arupconsult.com/algorithm/gender-affirming-hormone-therapy

to form close, supportive networks of friends that function equivalently to family units as "families of choice."[7]

Advance Care Planning

TGD adults may be particularly impacted by lack of advance care planning for end-of-life, with research showing that less than 5% of TGD individuals had completed a will or living will.[14]

Advance care planning should include additional emergency contacts, alternate decision makers, and who they would like their health information shared with. Given social networks may not be from families of origin, it is essential to complete advance directives to honor TGD patients' wishes and designate appropriate Power of Attorney (POA).

When older TGD adults are experiencing frailty, decline, or significant morbidity, end-of- life concerns may also emerge. Many aging TGD adults may fear not being able to care for themselves. In a national survey, palliative and hospice health care providers reported 21% had seen inadequate, disrespectful, or abusive care for TGD patients and 95% thought it likely that TGD patients delayed health care because of discrimination.[15] These findings underscore the importance of affirming care and connecting older TGD patients with affirming, culturally competent care.

Importantly, considerations to incorporate after-death care and affirmative end-of-life planning to ensure the sustained honor and respect of the patient's wishes postmortem will include funeral arrangements and memorial services in a manner concordant with the individual's identified gender. These preparations are fundamental in providing holistic and dignified care. The inclusion of these elements in advanced care planning guarantees the comprehensive preservation of the patient's dignity and wishes, both in life and after death.

Medication Review

As part of a CGA, patient's medication list should be reviewed at each visit with evaluation of need, risks, and medication interactions. This review process looks for the right medication at the right dose for the right condition.[10]

Tools to guide this process can include the Screening Tool of Older Persons Prescriptions and Screening Tool to Alert doctors to Right Treatment (STOPP/START) criteria, to provide guidance on avoiding potentially inappropriate medications, lack of adequate treatment, or omissions in older adults, in addition to referencing the Beers criteria for potentially inappropriate medication use. A patient-centered approach should be taken using shared decision-making with discussions about risks and benefits of each intervention and the patient's values and preferences, particularly when it comes to GAHT, where little evidence exists to guide starting or stopping therapy in older adults.

Sexual and Reproductive History

Sexual and reproductive history may be a sensitive topic for some TGD patients and, while important, this may be delayed until a safe and trusting relationship is established, unless immediately relevant.[3,5,7] For example, if patient presents with back pain, an in-depth sexual history/anatomic inventory is probably not appropriate and may exacerbate medical mistrust. All history should be approached through the trauma-informed care framework created by the Substance Abuse and Mental Health Services Administration (SAMHSA).

It is common for older adults to have been raised not to discuss or to hide their sexual desires and behaviors, especially if they were not in-line with traditional family values and relationships. The CDC's "Five P's" of sexual history may help provide a starting framework for safely discussing this topic, inquiring about partners, practices, sexually transmitted infection (STI) history, STI protection, and pregnancy plans.[15] The NCSH and National Lesbian, Gay, Bisexual, Transgender, Queer or Questioning, Intersex, Asexual (LGBTQIA) + Health Education Center have proposed adding a sixth P, recognizing that sexual pleasure is a factor in sexual behavior.

Several studies have shown that the burden of human immunodeficiency virus (HIV) and sexually transmitted infections (STIs) is high among transgender persons, especially transgender women and men who have sex with cisgender men.[5,7] Appropriate STI testing should be offered based on sexual behaviors and anatomy. Additionally, for people engaging in condomless sex, or other activities that increase acquisition of HIV, pre-exposure prophylaxis and post-exposure prophylaxis can be discussed. For more information on collecting a sexual history in older adults, please refer to the chapter on Preventative and Sexual Health of Older LGBTQ + Adults.

Anatomic Inventory

Older TGD patients may access gender-affirming hormonal and/or surgical interventions, or undergone procedures related to other conditions (eg, mastectomy due to cancer, or hysterectomy) that may influence screening recommendations. An anatomic or organ inventory allows the presence or absence of organs to be documented as well as any surgeries pertaining to those organs, which then can guide discussions for care, particularly for preventative health.

It is helpful to have a section in the medical chart that records what terms a patient uses to refer to their anatomy and then use that name or an agreed upon name during discussion.[16–18] This is a trauma-informed approach in what can be a sensitive, retraumatizing area for TGD older adults.

Clinicians should provide encouragement to do age-recommended health screening for each organ that is present.[4,17] The screening may come with some resistance as the patient may be uncomfortable talking about or even acknowledging that they have particular organs.

An example of how to broach this subject (provided by Dr Grasso) is "To provide you with the best clinical care, it is important for me to know if you have certain body parts. Is it okay if we talk through a list of body parts, and you can let me know whether you have these? If you use different words for parts of your body, please let me know."[18]

Cancer Screenings

Anatomy-based, rather than identity-based screenings are recommended for TGD patients.[4,9,17] As American College of Obstetrics and Gynecology notes "any anatomic structure present that warrants screening should be screened, regardless of gender identity."[17] All screening discussions and procedures should be approached in a trauma-informed framework.

Breast Cancer Screening

There are currently no evidence-based, TGD-specific breast cancer screening guidelines, which make a patient-centered discussion imperative. For transgender women who have breasts as a consequence of estrogen therapy, breast cancer screening should follow screening guidelines for cisgender women, as risk is elevated above cisgender men.[4] If transmasculine patients have not had chest reconstruction surgery or top surgery, it is recommended that providers apply the same breast cancer screening guidelines for cisgender women. In patients who have had chest or top surgery, the risk of breast cancer is significantly reduced. Mammography may be technically difficult due to the limited amount of residual breast tissue, however, other options, when indicated, include ultrasound or MRI. Clinicians should carefully document the patient's risk for breast cancer, including genetic risk, review the operative notes and surgical history to determine presence of residual tissue after mastectomy, and engage in shared decision-making about the need for breast cancer screening.

Cervical Cancer Screening

If a patient has a cervix, it is recommended they undergo cervical cancer screening in accordance with guidelines for cisgender women.[4,17] Due to the personal and intimate nature of the screening, it is quite common for the screening to cause dysphoria, which results in avoidance of the procedure.[3,4,7,9] Therefore, the patient should be approached with patience and understanding when discussing and planning for cervical cancer screenings. Options to encourage screening in a patient-centered approach include allowing patients to self-swab, and presence of a support person in the room. Human papillomavirus (HPV) swab samples self-collected by high-risk transmen had a sensitivity of 71.4% and a specificity of 98.2% in a study.[19] It is important to note that refusal of screening should not be a cause to withhold gender-affirming care. Additionally, testosterone therapy can cause atrophic changes to the cervix, which increases the likelihood of inadequate cytologic specimens, further reducing sensitivity of testing.

Ovarian Cancer Screening

Masculinizing regimens which include testosterone have not been shown to increase risk of ovarian cancer and prophylactic oophorectomy or screening is not required due to hormone use.

Endometrial Cancer Screening

For people with an endometrium, there is no evidence that testosterone-containing masculinizing regimens increase the risk of endometrial cancer; routine screening is not evidence based; although unexplained vaginal bleeding can occur, it remains abnormal and should be investigated.[20]

Testicular Cancer Screening

Feminizing regimens which include estrogen have not been shown to increase the risk of testicular cancer.

Prostate Cancer Screening

Routine prostate screening is complex and controversial. Just as with cisgender men, there should be shared decision-making with older transfeminine patients discussing harms and benefits in a patient-centered approach. Following vaginoplasty, transgender women will still have a prostate, which can be examined by palpating the anterior vaginal wall. GAHT decreases testosterone which overall reduces the risk for prostate cancer. However, although uncommon, transgender women can still develop prostate cancer and when they do, may have worse outcomes. PSA levels are unreliable when on 5 alpha reductase inhibitors, androgen blockers, or after gonadectomy. If serum PSA levels are tested, expert opinion states levels over 1 ng/mL require further investigation.[21]

Colorectal Cancer Screening

For colon cancer screening, follow routine colorectal cancer screening guidelines. If colorectal tissue is used to create a neovagina, this area can be examined via visual inspection during colonscopy.

Anal Cancer Screening

Per expert opinion, people living with human immunodeficiency virus (HIV), even when well-controlled, should follow best practice guidelines for anal cancer screening, including digital examination and anal pap smear for cytology. While anal pap smears for HIV-negative individuals are controversial, some experts recommend that anyone engaging in receptive anal intercourse and those who have had abnormal cervical cytology be screened.[22] Self-collected anal paps are feasible and may be preferred by patients, and increase adherence to screening guidelines.[22,23] There are no data on when to stop anal cancer screening, although like most cancer screening, cessation could be considered when life expectancy is less than 10 years.

Osteoporosis Screening

Regarding bone health, clinicians should discuss osteoporosis prevention measures, including active weight bearing exercise, healthy diet, and adequate calcium and vitamin D consumption. For osteoporosis screening, dual-energy X-ray absorptiometry scan for osteoporosis screening should be discussed with all TGD patients over the age of 65 regardless of status of gonadectomy or GAHT using a patient-centered approach.[4,9] WPATH recommends taking into account an individual's use of hormones, gonad status, and evaluation of osteoporosis risk factors in centering this discussion; gonadectomy and inconsistent use of GAHT could increase osteoporosis risk. Recent literature from the Netherlands found higher fracture risk in older transgender women over 50 when compared to age-matched cisgender men, at rates similar to cisgender women.[24] Overall, more research is needed in the field on bone health among TGD persons. It is important to note that gender-affirming hormone therapy is not associated with bone loss and may, in fact, restore or at least improve bone mineral density in TGD individuals.[25,26]

Smoking

Consistent with other populations that experience minority stress, TGD individuals have a higher prevalence of tobacco use.[4,7,26–28] As a result, they disproportionally experience the negative impact of tobacco use on health and wellbeing compared to cisgender populations.

All older TGD adults should undergo tobacco screenings and be offered appropriate behavioral and pharmacologic interventions to support decreased use with the goal of eventual cessation. Plans for interventions should include pathways to alleviate minority stress, and, if desired, incorporate gender-affirming care relevant to the patient's situation.[4,29]

Mental Health

Although limited, data from studies indicate TGD adults over 50 experience significantly higher rates of depressive symptoms than cisgender LGB and older heterosexual adults.[27,28] TGD adults are also more likely to attempt suicide than their cisgender LGB and older heterosexual adult counterparts; however, this does appear to decrease with age.[7,27] As previously stated, TGD older adults are also at a higher risk for social isolation and loss of support systems, which includes a lack of close friends and limited involvement of their family or children. When looking at older adult patients in general, literature shows those living with depression are likely to engage in excessive utilization of health care.[6,27]

In a report published by the National Center for Transgender Equality and National Gay and Lesbian Task Force in 2011, 41% of the respondents who identified as TGD reported attempting suicide (compared with 1.6% of the general population), 57% experienced "significant family rejection," and 19% experienced homelessness at some point in their lives due to being TGD.[7]

Screening for Depression and Anxiety

The United States Preventive Services Task Force recommends screening for depression for all adults. Older adults are less likely to bring up concerns about depression and anxiety to their PCP due to believing these feelings and behaviors are part of natural aging or character flaws.[8] There are several screening tools available, including the Patient Health Questionnaire (PHQ)-2/PHQ-9 and the Geriatric Depression Scale (GDS).[30]

For anxiety, the Generalized Anxiety Disorder 2-item (GAD-2)/GAD7-item (GAD-7) is widely used; the Geriatric Anxiety Inventory (GAI), like the GDS, was created specifically for older adults limiting somatic symptom evaluation. It can also be used in adults with mild cognitive impairment. It remains important to practice a trauma-informed approach and routinely screen older TGD adults given the high prevalence of mental health issues. This includes also screening for alcohol and substance use, which can occur at higher rates in TGD populations.

Primary Care for Gender-Affirming Hormone Therapy

Hormones may be provided as part of gender-affirming care. When provided under medical supervision, GAHT for adults is safe, effective, improves quality of life, and can be lifesaving.[26] The general goal is to create a hormonal environment, through manipulation of sex steroids that aligns with the patient's affirmed gender and their goals. There are some long-term risks and careful monitoring and screening is needed to reduce possible adverse events. It is imperative that the PCP knows what medications and dosing are being used and be knowledgeable about possible adverse reactions. For more information on gender affirming care, please refer to chapter 5.

Maintenance of Gender-Affirming Hormone Therapy

In general, GAHT is maintained throughout life for its desired masculinizing or feminizing effects. It is not known if doses of GAHT should be reduced as people age, although there are recommendations that estradiol should be given transdermally, rather than orally, to reduce the risk of venous thromboembolism in individuals aged 45 and over. There is documentation indicating that TGD individuals lose bone health when hormone therapy is discontinued, especially in individuals whose gonads have been removed.[11]

The current recommendations for individuals on GAHT include monitoring of sex steroid hormones levels every 3 months during the first year of hormone therapy or with any dose changes until stable dosing is achieved. After this, once or twice a year clinical evaluation and laboratory testing is recommended. For patients on testosterone, it is important that physicians check testosterone and hematocrit/hemoglobin levels. For patients receiving estrogens, it is important to check testosterone and estradiol levels. Additionally, electrolytes should also be monitored for patients who take spironolactone.

Patients should be carefully assessed whenever there are co-occurring conditions, such as cardiovascular disease (CVD) or hormonally responsive cancers that may be adversely impacted by GAHT. Patients with CVD will require optimization of traditional CV risk factors, including dyslipidemia, diabetes mellitus, hypertension, etc. Estrogen should be changed to a transdermal regimen if possible; however, no adjustments are recommended for testosterone treatment.[9,26] Patients with cancer should be evaluated by a multidisciplinary team and shared decision-making utilized to determine options, including whether to continue, reduce, change, or stop GAHT.

If the patient is planning to undergo gender-affirming surgery, it is important that the PCP collaborates with the patient's surgeon(s) regarding hormone use both before and after surgery.

SUMMARY

PCPs are often the initial contact point in the health care system for TGD patients who seek gender-affirming care. PCPs have a critical role to support older TGD patients, and advocate for them within the health care system. This necessitates that PCPs develop the knowledge and skills to deliver evidence-based, culturally appropriate care throughout the life-course. Clinicians should consider past and present gender-affirming interventions when applying preventive health guidelines. Care should be tailored to the unique experiences of TGD patients in order to promote overall health, wellbeing, and successful aging.

CLINICS CARE POINTS

- Create a safe, welcoming space for all patients.
- Use the patient's chosen pronouns and name.
- Review medications at each visit.
- Sexual and reproductive history conversations using trauma-informed framework ensure appropriate care.
- Recommend age-appropriate health screening that is anatomy based for each organ present.
- TGD care mirrors geriatric care, with recommended CGA at initiation of care and subsequent visits, inclusive of the 4 M's with some transgender-specific geriatric needs.
- Smoking screening, coupled with education and cessation resources, should be discussed.
- Mental health screening and follow-up should be addressed at each visit.
- Any physician who has gained basic competencies in transgender health can start hormones once GAHT is deemed appropriate, with a patient-centered discussion and sharing of expectations for treatment prior to initiation.
- Monitoring of GAHT should include serum sex hormone levels, and hematocrit and electrolytes if indicated

ACKNOWLEDGMENTS

The author would like to acknowledge Kris Chen's contributions to the writing of this article. His expertise in content, proofreading, and editorial suggestions, and support was invaluable.

DISCLOSURE

Authors have no financial disclosures.

FUNDING

Dr Radix is supported by the National Institute of Mental Health under award number R25MH087217. Dr Chen is not funded.

REFERENCES

1. Terms and Tips. Oregon Health & Science University Transgender Health Program. Available at: https://www.ohsu.edu/transgender-health/transgender-health-program-terms-and-tips. Accessed October 1, 2023.
2. Glossary of Term: Transgender. GLAAD Media Reference Guide 11th ed. Available at: https://glaad.org/reference/trans-terms/. Accessed October 1, 2023.
3. Scheim AI, Baker KE, Restar AJ, et al. Health and health care among transgender adults in the United States. Annu Rev Publ Health 2022;43(1):503–23.
4. Coleman E, Radix AE, Bouman WP, et al. Standards of Care for the Health of Transgender and Gender Diverse People. Int J Transgend Health 2022; 23(Suppl 1):S1–259.
5. Fredriksen-Goldsen KI. Resilience and disparities among Lesbian, Gay, Bisexual, and transgender older adults. Public Policy Aging Rep 2011;21(3):3–7.
6. Shiu C, Kim HJ, Fredriksen-Goldsen K. Health care Engagement among LGBT older adults: the role of depression diagnosis and Symptomatology. Gerontol 2017;57(suppl 1):S105–14.
7. Grant JM, Mottet LA, Tanis J, et al. Injustice at every turn: A report of the National Transgender Discrimination Survey. National Center for Transgender Equality and National Gay and Lesbian Task Force; Washington, DC Feb 2011. Available at: https://transequality.org/sites/default/files/docs/resources/NTDS_Report.pdf. Accessed October 1, 2023
8. Corrigan PW, Druss BG, Perlick DA. The impact of mental illness stigma on seeking and Participating in mental health care. Psychol Sci Publ Interest 2014;15(2):37–70.
9. Gamble RM, Taylor SS, Huggins AD, et al. Trans-specific Geriatric Health Assessment (TGHA): an inclusive clinical guideline for the geriatric transgender patient in a primary care setting. Maturitas 2020;132:70–5.
10. Mate K, Fulmer T, Pelton L, et al. Evidence for the 4Ms: Interactions and outcomes across the care Continuum. J Aging Health 2021;33(7–8):469–81.
11. Unger CA. Hormone therapy for transgender patients. Transl Androl Urol 2016; 5(6):877–84.
12. Foley M. Herbal Medicine for Gender Euphoria. The Alchemist's Kitchen. Available at: https://wisdom.thealchemistskitchen.com/?s=gender+euphoria. Accessed October 1, 2023.
13. Midnight, D. Holistic Health for Transgender & Gender Variant Folks. Transgender Herbal Care. Available at: https://www.berkeleyherbalcenter.org/wp-content/uploads/2020/05/Midnight_D_Transgender_Care.pdf. Accessed October 1, 2023.
14. Witten TM. End of life, chronic illness, and trans-identities. J Soc Work End Life Palliat Care 2014;10(1):34–58.
15. Stein GL, Berkman C, O'Mahony S, et al. Experiences of Lesbian, Gay, Bisexual, and transgender patients and families in hospice and palliative care: Perspectives of the palliative care team. J Palliat Med 2020 Jun;23(6):817–24.
16. Centers for Disease Control and Prevention, STI and HIV Infection Risk Assessment. Sexually Transmitted Infections Treatment Guidelines, 2021. Available at: www.cdc.gov/std/treatment-guidelines/clinical-risk.htm. Accessed October 1, 2023.
17. Health care for transgender and gender diverse individuals. ACOG Committee opinion No. 823. American College of Obstetricians and Gynecologists. Obstet Gynecol 2021;137:e75–88.

18. Grasso C, Goldhammer H, Thompson J, et al. Optimizing gender-affirming medical care through anatomical inventories, clinical decision support, and population health management in electronic health record systems. J Am Med Inf Assoc 2021;28(11):2531–5.
19. Reisner SL, Deutsch MB, Peitzmeier SM, et al. Test performance and acceptability of self- versus provider-collected swabs for high-risk HPV DNA testing in female-to-male trans masculine patients. PLoS One 2018;13(3):e0190172.
20. Grimstad FW, Fowler KG, New EP, et al. Uterine pathology in transmasculine persons on testosterone: a retrospective multicenter case series. Am J Obstet Gynecol 2019;220(3):257.e1–7.
21. Nik-Ahd F, Jarjour A, Figueiredo J, et al. Prostate-specific Antigen screening in transgender patients. Eur Urol 2023;83(1):48–54.
22. Hirsch BE, McGowan JP, Fine SM, et al. Screening for Anal Dysplasia and Cancer in Adults With HIV. Johns Hopkins University; 2022 Aug 9. Available at: https://www.ncbi.nlm.nih.gov/books/NBK556472/. Assessed October 1, 2023.
23. Chin-Hong PV, Berry JM, Cheng SC, et al. Comparison of patient- and clinician-collected anal cytology samples to screen for human papillomavirus-associated anal intraepithelial neoplasia in men who have sex with men. Ann Intern Med 2008;149(5):300–6.
24. Wiepjes CM, de Blok CJ, Staphorsius AS, et al. Fracture risk in trans women and trans men using long-term gender-affirming hormonal treatment: a Nationwide Cohort study. J Bone Miner Res 2020 Jan;35(1):64–70.
25. Giacomelli G, Meriggiola MC. Bone health in transgender people: a narrative review. Therapeutic Advances in Endocrinology and Metabolism 2022;13. https://doi.org/10.1177/20420188221099346.
26. Asscheman H, Giltay EJ, Megens JA, et al. A long-term follow-up study of mortality in transsexuals receiving treatment with cross-sex hormones. Eur J Endocrinol 2011;164(4):635–42.
27. Fredriksen-Goldsen KI, Cook-Daniels L, Kim HJ, et al. Physical and mental health of transgender older adults: an at-risk and underserved population. Gerontologist 2014;54(3):488–500.
28. The Population Research in Identities and Disparities for Equality (PRIDE) Study. Available at: https://pridestudy.org/research. Accessed September 1, 2023.
29. Pachankis JEA. Transdiagnostic minority stress treatment approach for Gay and Bisexual Men's Syndemic health conditions. Arch Sex Behav 2016;44:1843–60.
30. Maurer DM, Raymond TJ, Davis BN. Depression: screening and diagnosis. Am Fam Physician 2018;98(8):508–15.

Human Immunodeficiency Virus in Older Adults

Matthew L. Russell, MD, MSc[a,*], Amy Justice, MD, PhD[b]

KEYWORDS

• HIV • Aging • LGBTQIA • Geriatric syndromes

KEY POINTS

- Older individuals are at substantially increased risk of delayed diagnosis and treatment of HIV.
- Currently, over half of the population of people living with HIV (PWH) are aged 50 years and over and this is expected to increase to 70% by the year 2030.
- PWH are exposed to the combined effects of age-related diseases and the extended impact of HIV and its treatment.
- Even among those with suppressed virus, HIV causes chronic inflammation substantially increasing the individual's risk of many aging-associated conditions.

INTRODUCTION

Before combination therapy for HIV infection became available in the late 1990s, life expectancy after an AIDS diagnosis was measured in months. Combination antiretroviral therapy (ART) now allows people with HIV (PWH) to age, often living several decades after diagnosis. However, aging with HIV is different than aging without HIV. PWH are exposed to the combined effects of age-related diseases and the extended impact of HIV and its treatment. Many PWH also continue to smoke, drink alcohol, and use cannabis and other substances as they age, further complicating the aging process. Prolonged HIV infection, multimorbidity, polypharmacy, and multi-substance use, all increase susceptibility to age-related conditions and to adverse effects of medication. As a result, PWH are experiencing earlier onset of geriatric syndromes including cognitive compromise, falls and fractures, and frailty.

Further, marginalized populations have been afflicted with HIV to a greater extent than the general population and experience ongoing challenges accessing ART, and more general medical and psychiatric care. LGBTQIA PWH are often members of multiple stigmatized marginalized groups. A diagnosis of HIV infection often adds to this stigma which may impede appropriate geriatric care.

[a] Harvard University, Massachusetts General Hospital, 55 Fruit Street, Yawkey 2C, Boston, MA 02114, USA; [b] Department of General Internal Medicine, Yale School of Medicine, Yale University, 950 Campbell Avenue, West Haven, CT 06516, USA
* Corresponding author.
E-mail address: mlrussell@mgh.harvard.edu

Clin Geriatr Med 40 (2024) 285–298
https://doi.org/10.1016/j.cger.2023.12.004
geriatric.theclinics.com
0749-0690/24/

DEMOGRAPHICS

Currently, over half of the population of people living with HIV (PWH) are aged 50 years and over and this is expected to increase to 70% by the year 2030.[1] Older men of color and men who have sex with men are disproportionately impacted by HIV.[2] Although most older adults were diagnosed with HIV at earlier ages, older adults are less likely to undergo HIV testing, and this can lead to delayed diagnosis and presenting at later stages of HIV infection.[3]

The life expectancy of HIV-infected individuals has improved dramatically with the advent of ART and more people are living with HIV than ever before. In 1996, a 20-year-old with HIV was expected to live an additional 19.1 years. In 2011, that number increased to 53 years.[4] Despite ART, there is still an 8-to-11-year gap in life expectancy between HIV-infected and non-infected populations.[4,5] It is important to note that PWH aged 50 years and over account for 70% of deaths among PWH.[4] Moreover, the primary causes of death for those with access to ART combination treatments are chronic diseases such as cancer, cardiovascular disease, and cognitive impairment.[6]

HIV infection is associated with 1 to 5 years earlier onset of several chronic conditions including cardiovascular disease, dyslipidemia, diabetes mellitus, chronic kidney disease, chronic obstructive pulmonary disease (COPD), psychiatric disorders, and some cancers.[7] In addition, PWH demonstrate multimorbidity, polypharmacy, frailty and other geriatric syndromes including falls, depression, cognitive impairment, and risk of malnutrition at higher rates than HIV-negative individuals in age-matched studies.[8]

Delayed Diagnosis

Between 2015 and 2019, there was a 15% increase in incidence of HIV among people 50 years and older, the largest increases of any age group in the United States.[9] Concerningly, in nearly half the cases, diagnosis was delayed (CD4 cell count <350 cells/μL) in this age group.[10] Compared with people less than 50 years, those 50 years of age and older are two to four times more likely to have their HIV diagnosis delayed. Of note, the optimal window for diagnosis may be shorter for older individuals because CD4 counts decline naturally with age and HIV accentuates risk of age-associated comorbid disease.[11]

With increased life expectancy, older adults are continuing to enjoy sexual activity[12,13] and may also continue to use alcohol and other substances.[14,15] Substance use, age-associated erectile dysfunction, and women being beyond child-bearing age all contribute to inconsistent use of condoms,[16,17] increasing opportunities for HIV transmission. This is particularly concerning because older PWH have delayed presentation for HIV treatment compared with younger PWH, prolonging the period in which they have detectable virus and may expose others to infection. Delayed presentation also decreases their ability to benefit from early ART initiation.[18,19]

We recommend HIV screening in high-risk older adults. This includes self-testing to empower older individuals to learn their HIV status and seek care. We recommend providers to have routine clinical discussion of sexual health and substance use to identify those at highest risk, improved response to early HIV indicator conditions (persistent influenza-like symptoms, bacterial pneumonia, herpes zoster, lymphocytopenia, thrombocytopenia, and cervical or vulvar dysplasia), use of electronic decision support to prompt and facilitate HIV testing, and more widespread use of pre-exposure prophylaxis (PrEP), possibly on-demand PrEP, among those at high risk.

PATHOPHYSIOLOGY

Human Immunodeficiency Virus Infection

HIV attaches to and penetrates host cells via CD4+ molecules and chemokine receptors and subsequently integrates into the host genome. HIV specifically targets and infects CD4+ lymphocytes leading to their depletion and subsequent cellular immune deficiency. This leads to increased susceptibility to opportunistic infection and neoplasms. HIV infection leads to chronic inflammation. HIV infection with long-term effective ART is associated with a serum inflammatory signature, including markers of inflammasome activation, and an increased activation of monocytes on inflammasome stimulation.[20] Although combination ART is remarkably successful at suppressing the virus, it does not eradicate it. Even among those with suppressed virus, HIV causes chronic inflammation increasing the individual's risk of many aging associated conditions.

HIV-infected individuals have been noted to have higher prevalence of cardiovascular disease, cancer, osteopenia/osteoporosis, liver disease, sexual dysfunction, hearing deficit, sleep disorders, falls, and cognitive complaints when compared with matched controls.[21] Several factors likely contribute to this risk, in addition to the chronic inflammation associated with HIV infection, including ART side-effects, polypharmacy, increased physiologic frailty, and the aging of the immune system itself.[22]

Human immunodeficiency virus and geriatric principles: The 5 Ms

Using the 5 Ms framework conceptualized by Tinetti and colleagues, many of the challenges experienced by PWH can be delineated using this model.[23] This framework includes evaluation of a person's medication management, mobility, mentation, expression of what matters most, and an appreciation of multi-complexity. The pressing challenges for PWH under the multi-complexity heading including isolation, trauma, substance abuse, housing insecurity.

Medication management

Principles of Human Immunodeficiency Virus medication management The advent of triple drug combination ART in 1997 revolutionized the care of people with HIV infection and made aging with HIV possible. The underlying principle was to attack viral replication at multiple points in the cycle, thereby requiring simultaneous use of different drug classes. This approach proved highly effective at suppressing the virus enabling nearly everyone taking the regimen to attain complete viral suppression.

Polypharmacy PWH with access to combination ART are living longer and developing multiple chronic conditions requiring non-ART medications. Defined as concurrent use of five or more chronic medications, polypharmacy, is associated with adverse drug events, potentially inappropriate medications, falls, cognitive impairments, mortality, and hospitalization.[24–26] Polypharmacy and associated adverse outcomes are a particular problem for PWH, who typically cross the threshold for polypharmacy 10 years earlier than people without HIV and have greater physiologic frailty making them more susceptible to the harms of polypharmacy.[27–30] Thus, it is highly desirable to consider non-medication-based therapies for bothersome symptoms and comorbid conditions when possible.

Drug–drug interactions ART medications commonly interact with non-ART medications.[31] For example, boosted regimens, including protease inhibitors and the early integrase strand transfer inhibitor elvitegravir–cobicistat, can increase drug concentrations and the risk of adverse effects of co-medications via inhibition of CYP3A4 and its transporters.[32] Interactions between ART and non-ART medications are associated with hospitalization after adjusting for CD4 cell count, protease inhibitor-based regimen, substance use, and non-ART medication count.[31,33] Although now being prescribed less frequently, the use of boosted regimens remains common.[34]

Across a range of commonly observed medication counts, known drug interactions are five to six times more common in real-world data than if medications are randomly selected. This higher number of interactions is probably because medications that are given to address specific health conditions have overlapping mechanisms and adverse events. This is particularly true for PWH, most likely because ART medications have an exceptionally large number of drug–drug interactions.[32,35]

This is problematic for three reasons. First, as people age, they become more susceptible to the harmful effects of these substances. Second, people aging with HIV are physiologically even more susceptible than their age-matched uninfected counterparts. Third, continued substance use of alcohol and other drugs interacts in important ways with polypharmacy, increasing the likelihood of adverse effects from medications.

Mentation

Interface between human immunodeficiency virus-associated diseases and age-associated cognitive disease Earlier in the epidemic, before widespread availability of triple-drug combination therapy, HIV-associated neurocognitive disorder was commonplace. However, because ART became widely used, it is rarely observed. Now the major drivers of cognitive difficulties include polypharmacy, substance use, and neurovascular disease. Of these, polypharmacy and substance use are the most immediately modifiable. For example, a recent study demonstrated that the risk of delirium is greater among those aging with HIV than uninfected age-matched comparators and that both groups experienced higher rates of delirium associated with anticholinergic medications, non-anticholinergic neurocognitively active medications, and level of ongoing alcohol consumption[27]

Cognitive screening The US Preventive Services Task Force (USPSTF) has found insufficient evidence to recommend or against screening for cognitive impairment in older adults in the general population in the absence of known impairments.[36] Thus, screening should be based on symptomatology.

The Montreal Cognitive Assessment (MoCA) is available online and is a validated instrument that is available in many languages to screen for mild cognitive impairments. Because of variable quality in testing, in 2019, fee-based training and certification through MoCA cognition became required to administer the MoCA.[37] The MoCA takes approximately 10 to 15 minutes to administer and consists of 30 items that measure function in eight cognitive domains.[38] A score of 26 points or lower (out of a maximum of 30) indicates cognitive impairment. The MoCA has been found to be more sensitive than the mini-mental status examination (MMSE) at detecting mild cognitive impairment in the general population.[39,40] The Rowland University Dementia Assessment Scale (RUDAS) is another cognitive screening tool that has been studied in cross-cultural populations and has been validated as a screen for dementia especially in those with lower levels of literacy.[41] This tool is free to use at present. Unlike the MMSE, the RUDAS did not seem to be impacted by gender, education, or language.[42]

Mobility. Under the general category of mobility, we focus on ensuring that a person is functionally able to do for themselves not only in basic terms but also in more complex ways such that they are able to accomplish what is important to them. Frailty, fall risk assessment, and bone health are key factors in the comprehensive geriatrics assessment.

Frailty and human immunodeficiency virus Frailty is defined as a clinically recognizable state of increased vulnerability resulting from aging-associated decline in reserve and function across multiple physiologic systems such that the ability to cope with every day or acute stressors is compromised.[43] Frailty has been characterized clinically by Fried and colleagues as meeting three out of five phenotypic criteria: low grip strength, low energy, slowed walking speed, low physical activity, and/or unintentional weight loss. One critique of the Fried frailty score is that it does not consider cognitive, mental health, and sensory status. The frailty index[44] is a more comprehensive deficit-based scoring but even that may not capture the additional elements of frailty including trauma, isolation, and insecure housing issues that are experienced by PWH at rates much higher than the general population. In addition, resulting physiologic frailty or the amount of remaining organ system reserve has been reproducibly measured using the Veterans Aging Cohort Study Index (VACS Index). The VACS Index is more predictive of mortality, hospitalization, cognitive compromise, falls, fractures, and biologic measures of aging than these other measures.[27,44–47]

Measured in many ways, frailty is associated with a decreased quality of life, hospitalizations, and a greater risk of mortality.[46] Frailty has been strongly associated with poorly controlled HIV infection.[48] PWH can experience frailty at higher rates than age-matched noninfected individuals.[49] Frailty in this population has been associated with increasing age, greater comorbidity, longer duration of known HIV infection and ART, history of AIDS, and low nadir and current CD4 T cell count.[50] Moreover, frailty is inversely related to successful cognitive aging in PWH.[51] As listed below, both pre-frailty and frailty are quite prevalent in cognitively impaired PWH aged 60 years and over.[8] PWH can experience deficits in activities of daily living at higher rates than noninfected individuals.[52] In older adults with HIV, there are several findings that raise concern for impaired mobility (**Fig. 1**).

PWH can experience an assortment of challenges that can amplify the syndrome of frailty. Frailty in HIV patients often overlaps with geriatric syndromes and conditions, such as cognitive impairment, sensory deficits, falls, and polypharmacy.[8] These factors need to be considered when designing treatment strategies.

The International Conference of Frailty and Sarcopenia Research developed clinical practice guidelines, one of which is to screen for frailty in adults aged 65 years and older using a validated screening tool.[53] The recognition of similarities in the biology and clinical phenotype between older adults and HIV-infected adults led to the study of frailty in HIV.[48] For PWH, there is no consensus on the best tool to assess for frailty.

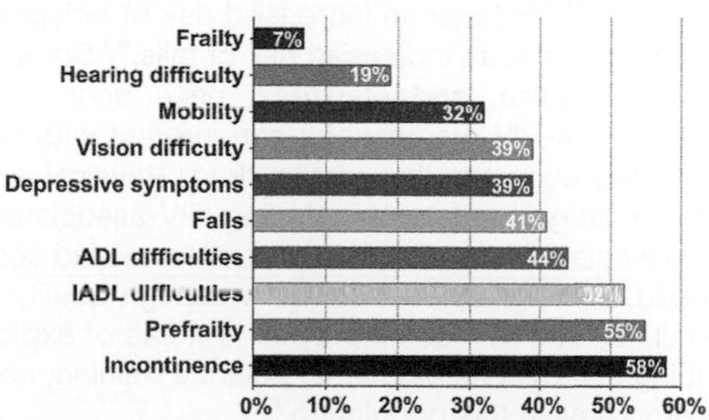

Fig. 1. Frequencies of geriatric syndromes among older HIV-infected adults with mild neurocognitive disorder (MND). (*From* Hosaka, K. R. J., Greene, M., Premeaux, T. A., Javandel, S., Allen, I. E., Ndhlovu, L. C., & Valcour, V. (2019). Geriatric Syndromes in Older Adults Living with HIV and Cognitive Impairment. Journal of the American Geriatrics Society, 67(9), 1913–1916. https://doi.org/10.1111/jgs.16034.)

In much HIV research on this issue, the Fried frailty phenotype is used. Another frailty tool is the VACS Index, and this has an online calculator available.[2]

The frailty index, a cumulative deficit-based index, has also been used, although implementation of this tool outside of a comprehensive geriatric assessment visit can be burdensome.[54] In clinical practice, the challenge is to screen for and recognize frailty and, if present, refer for a comprehensive geriatric assessment.[55] This puts the geriatrics provider in a unique position to evaluate and impact the functional status of individuals who are chronologically younger than the population they typically serve but are biologically older. Frailty assessments in PWH should consider the unique considerations of HIV. Frailty may impact the ability to attend medical appointments, comply with complex medication regimens, and adhere to other recommendations such as outpatient physical therapy and optimized diet. Attaining virologic suppression through ART has been shown to decrease the prevalence of frailty.

As with other models of addressing frailty, the use of multi-disciplinary and nonpharmacologic interventions for PWH experiencing frailty is key.[56] To combat frailty, increased exercise, optimized nutrition, reduction of polypharmacy, and evaluation and treatment of fall risk in PWH aged 50 years and over are common recommendations. Additional evaluation for social determinants that can impact frailty risk should be done as well. This includes assessment of economic and educational status, social and community connections, neighborhood/housing, and access to health care.[57]

Falls and human immunodeficiency virus A third of people aged 65 years and older experience a fall on an annual basis.[58] HIV-infected adults may be at a higher risk of sustaining an injurious fall or fracture due to low bone density, sarcopenia, neuropathy, cognitive impairment, and frailty.[59] The fall rate in middle-aged PWH (45–65 years) is like the fall rate reported for all US adults aged 65 years and older at 25% to 30%.[59] PWH lose bone mass at an accelerated rate than noninfected controls and can be diagnosed with low bone mineral density at earlier ages.[60] As a geriatric syndrome, the etiology of a fall is multifactorial and requires an appreciation of all potential contributors. In addition, falls result in substantial morbidity and poor health outcomes.[61] In one study, sociodemographic and HIV-related factors were significantly associated with falls. These include socioeconomic status, relationship and living status, and a self-reported AIDS diagnosis.[62]

As with all fall-related events, the workup should include a thorough assessment of a patient's medication and substance use history. Benzodiazepines, psychotropics, alcohol, and other recreational drugs can increase the risk of falls due to impact on balance and coordination. PWH have an increased risk of polypharmacy and drug-drug interactions putting them at an increased risk of falls.[63] Some ART medications, including didanosine, stavudine, and efavirenz, have been associated with an increased risk of falls.[59] Non-HIV medications can interact with HIV medications to potentiate or diminish the concentration of the drug. Physical examination should include evaluation for sensory impairment including HIV-associated polyneuropathy. Assessment for HIV-associated neurodegenerative disease and cognitive impairment should also be checked. Although there is currently no high-quality evidence for interventions to reduce fall risk in PWH, some proposed areas of exploration include the impact of deprescribing high-risk medications, balance training, home safety evaluations, and exercise programs in this population.[60]

Bone health and human immunodeficiency virus HIV infection as well as some HIV medications including tenofovir disoproxil fumarate and some protease inhibitors may increase the risk of bone loss in people with HIV.[64] Low bone mineral density is prevalent in PWH.[65] In one study, the prevalence of osteoporosis in PWH was noted to be three times higher than that of non-HIV-infected control subjects, particularly in those receiving ART. In one study of HIV-infected individuals, the prevalence of osteopenia was 36% and osteoporosis was 4%. The median age in this study was 43 years of age.[66] The causes of low bone density in HIV are multifactorial and are due to interplay between HIV infection, usual osteoporosis risk factors, high rates of tobacco and alcohol use, low vitamin D levels, and ART-related processes. The prevalence of vitamin D deficiency is high in PWH with observation of 36.8% for mild and 10% for severe vitamin D deficiency in one study[67] ART naïve individuals have a high prevalence of osteopenia suggesting that viremia can impact bone density likely through inflammatory pathways. HIV proteins increase osteoclast activity. Hypogonadism and low dietary calcium intake are other contributors.

The USPSTF recommends bone density screening (BMD) for women aged 65 years and older.[2] The National Osteoporosis Foundation also recommends screening for men aged 70 years and older as well as in postmenopausal women and men aged 50 years and over who experience a fracture.[68] By extrapolation, those with HIV are recommended to have BMD checked at age 50 years and over because additional risk factors and osteopenia are already quite prevalent.[69]

Matters most

Ensuring patient-centered care In the medical management of older adults, ensuring that patients are receiving care in line with their expressed goals is a cornerstone of geriatric clinical care. Much of the work done in this area centers on eliciting these goals and ensuring patient autonomy even when decision-making capacity is lost. Eliciting these goals involves engaging the patient in discussions of priorities, and having frank conversations about planning for aging, decline, and death. This includes identifying and informing a health care proxy of their wishes and values. PWH may have struggled with trauma, alienation, mental illness, and stigma even before they graduated into older adult status,[70] and they may have strong feelings about how and where care is provided as well as what is shared and with whom. The many medical appointments and coordination with subspecialists can leave patients in a state of perpetual medicalization which can interfere with quality of life. Earlier onset of chronic conditions and geriatric syndromes can add to the complexity of talking about what matters most especially if it means requiring assistance in the home or transition to a more supportive living environment. The double stigma of aging and HIV[71] can be compounded further by the stigma against people from sexual minorities. Helping patients navigate their care in a way that ensures their autonomy and maximizes their comfort and trust is key.

PWH can experience the usual challenges of aging with additional factors added in. Specifically, there can be unmet basic needs. These can include access to food and clothing as well as housing-related costs and the risk of homelessness.[72] Housing that is affordable and accessible (for functionally impaired older PWH) is necessary and many PWH have experienced stigma related to their HIV and sexuality. Housing needs to be both accessible and safe/welcoming.

Multi-complexity: special considerations for people with human immunodeficiency virus

Isolation The absence of a partner increases the risk of negative outcomes.[73] Many PWH may also experience isolation from families of origin for any number of reasons. Frailty and subsequent limitations in mobility can impose additional risk of isolation. Older lesbian, gay, bisexual, transgender, queer, intersex, and asexual (LGBTQIA) people with HIV face increased risk of isolation and loneliness. In a study of HIV-positive adults aged 50 years and older, 58% reported any loneliness symptoms, with 24% reporting mild, 22% moderate, and 12% severe loneliness. Social isolation and loneliness are associated with poor self-rated physical health and depression and increased risk of mortality.[74] Risk factors for isolation include estrangement from families of origin, loss of friends to AIDS, and societal barriers that could have interfered with forming life partnerships. In addition, LGBTQIA older adults are more likely to be single and live alone and less likely to have children than their heterosexual peers. Fear of discrimination can lead LGBTQ + older adults avoid asking for help. The concept of "re-entering the closet" is a stressor that can act as a barrier to accessing supports specifically designed to address loneliness.[75]

Substance use A study of HIV-positive men aged 50 years and older in New York City revealed that 53% of men reported regular alcohol use, 21.4% used inhaled nitrites ("poppers"), and 22.9% reported hard drug use (crystal methamphetamine, cocaine, crack, heroin, ecstasy, gamma hydroxybutyrate (GHB), ketamine, and/or lysergic acid diethylamide (LSD) or phencyclidine (PCP). Twenty-eight percent reported marijuana use.[76] In addition to the associated health risks associated with each substance, there are other factors for the geriatric provider to consider. One is ongoing counseling regarding reducing risky sexual behavior and coinfection with other sexually transmitted infections (STIs) and viruses because of concurrent drug use. Stigma related to ongoing drug use is a risk factor for disengaging with care and ART noncompliance. Many PWH have experienced trauma throughout their lives. Patient-centered trauma-informed care is a cornerstone for partnering with PWH.[77]

The current generation of people aging in the United States is much more likely to continue to use substances, most especially tobacco and marijuana.[78] Those aging with HIV are even more likely to do so. There is a high prevalence (27%) of hazardous alcohol use (defined as AUDIT-C score[79] greater than 4) in PLWH. Hazardous alcohol use was more prevalent in subjects who reported current illicit drug use including cocaine/crack and marijuana use. This has implications on outcomes of PWH including maintaining viral suppression through adherence to ART and overall survival. Older adults with HIV had a lower prevalence of hazardous alcohol use than their younger coundterparts, although alcohol use in this demographic was still substantial.[80]

The rate of marijuana use among PWH is higher than the general population with 77% of PWH reporting lifetime cannabis use compared with uninfected population (44.5%). This trend was noted in both past year and past month use as well. Forty-two percent of PWH more than age 50 years report current use of marijuana.[81] With growing social acceptance and legalization of marijuana, many PWH use marijuana not just for recreation but also for treatment of some common conditions including pain, anxiety, depression, nausea, and anorexia.[82] The current use of marijuana is associated with less than 100% compliance with ART and missed visits.[82] On the other hand, research has been done looking at the impact of cannabis use on reduction of peripheral inflammatory markers in HIV.[83]

Recent methamphetamine use in sexual minority populations is two to four times that of the general population. This is even more pronounced in urban areas with high concentrations of sexual minority men.[84] Methamphetamine use in PWH can impact ART compliance, mood, and lead to suboptimal viral load and increased risk of onward transmission of HIV.[85]

Care models With increased survival, patients with HIV are occupying a unique space in health care delivery. From an infectious disease standpoint, the modern goals for basic HIV care are early diagnosis, connection to health care, early initiation of combination

ART with good adherence, and the attainment of viral suppression. As most PWH are aged 50 years and over, they are experiencing earlier and more intense onset of chronic conditions and geriatric syndromes. The care model must become more nuanced.

To address this, several models of care delivery have been assessed: an outpatient referral or consultation to the geriatrician, combined HIV and geriatric multispecialty clinic, and dually trained providers within one clinical setting. One major piece of patient feedback especially for PWH between age 50 and 60 years is the perceived stigma of seeing a geriatrician. The moniker alone was enough to dissuade patients from attending. The combined clinic provided "one stop shopping" for PWH. On the one hand, this was an opportunity for the geriatric skill set to reach the patient in a trusted environment with other familiar faces. On the other hand, replication of this model proved to be financially onerous as the most successful programs are maintained by philanthropic donations. Last, the dual-trained provider is an outstanding resource and is extremely scarce. Overlying all these models is the locus of clinical control. Many patients express feeling lost in a sea of specialists and health care providers. Finding ways to ensure that there are clear lines of delegation and collaboration is key to any successful model.

SUMMARY

People aging with HIV can experience additional health challenges when compared with their noninfected counterparts. The advent of ART has allowed people to survive long enough to experience age-associated chronic conditions and geriatric syndromes, many of which PWH experience at an earlier age. Engaging this population through the lens of a geriatric perspective can assist primary care and infectious disease providers in adapting their practices to ensure that their unique needs can be assessed and addressed.

CLINICS CARE POINTS

- Older individuals are at substantially increased risk of delayed diagnosis and treatment of HIV.
- Currently, over half of the population of people living with HIV (PWH) are aged 50 years and over and this is expected to increase to 70% by the year 2030.
- PWH are exposed to the combined effects of age-related diseases and the extended impact of HIV and its treatment.
- Even among those with suppressed virus, HIV causes chronic inflammation substantially increasing the individual's risk of many aging-associated conditions.

DISCLOSURE

Dr M.L. Russell reports no commercial or financial conflicts of interest. He is a Grant Recipient from U.S. Department of Health and Human Services, United States (HHS) Office of Infectious Disease and HIV/AIDS Policy (OIDP) and the Administration for Community Living, United States (ACL) "Innovations for Needs of People Aging with HIV/Long-Term Survivors in Urban Communities" Challenge. Justice reports no commercial or financial conflicts of interest. She is a grant recipient from the National Institutes of Health, United States and the United States Veterans Affairs Office of Research Development.

REFERENCES

1. Wing E. The aging population with HIV infection. Trans Am Clin Climatol Assoc 2017;131–44.
2. https://www.hiv.gov/hiv-basics/overview/data-and-trends/impact-on-racial-and-ethnic-minorities/.
3. Youssef E, Wright J, Delpech V, et al. Factors associated with testing for HIV in people aged ≥50 years: a qualitative study. BMC Publ Health 2018;18(1):1204.
4. Marcus JL, Chao CR, Leyden WA, et al. Narrowing the gap in life expectancy between hiv-infected and hiv-uninfected individuals with access to care. J Acquir Immune Defic Syndr 2016;39–46.
5. Marcus JL, Leyden WA, Alexeeff SE, et al. Comparison of overall and comorbidity-free life expectancy between insured adults with and without HIV infection, 2000-2016. JAMA Netw Open 2020;3(6):e207954.
6. Deeks SG, Lewin SR, Havlir DV. The end of AIDS: HIV infection as a chronic disease. Lancet 2013;382(9903):1525–33.
7. Serrano-Villar S, Gutiérrez F, Miralles C, et al. Human immunodeficiency virus as a chronic disease: evaluation and management of nonacquired immune deficiency syndrome-defining conditions. Open Forum Infect Dis 2016;3(2). https://doi.org/10.1093/ofid/ofw097.
8. Hosaka KRJ GM, Premeaux TA, Javandel S, et al. Geriatric syndromes in older adults living with HIV and cognitive impairment. J Am Geriatr Soc 2019;67(9):1913–6.
9. Prevention CfDCa. Estimated HIV incidence and prevalence in the United States, 2015-2019. Vol. 26. 2021. HIV Surveillance Supplemental Report.
10. Justice AC, Goetz MB, Stewart CN, et al. Delayed presentation of HIV among older individuals: a growing problem. Lancet HIV 2022;9(4):e269–80.
11. Montano M, Oursler KK, Xu K, et al. Biological ageing with HIV infection: evaluating the geroscience hypothesis. Lancet Healthy Longev 2022;3(3):e194–205.
12. Lindau ST, Gavrilova N. Sex, health, and years of sexually active life gained due to good health: evidence from two US population based cross sectional surveys of ageing. BMJ 2010;340:c810.
13. Nicolosi A, Buvat J, Glasser DB, et al. Sexual behaviour, sexual dysfunctions and related help seeking patterns in middle-aged and elderly Europeans: the global study of sexual attitudes and behaviors. World J Urol 2006;24(4):423–8.
14. Collaborators GBDA. Alcohol use and burden for 195 countries and territories, 1990-2016: a systematic analysis for the global burden of disease study 2016. Lancet 2018;392(10152):1015–35.
15. Kuerbis A. Substance use among older adults: an update on prevalence, etiology, assessment, and intervention. Gerontology 2020;66(3):249–58.
16. Ehrenstein V, Horton NJ, Samet JH. Inconsistent condom use among HIV-infected patients with alcohol problems. Drug Alcohol Depend 2004;73(2):159–66.
17. Schick V, Herbenick D, Reece M, et al. Sexual behaviors, condom use, and sexual health of Americans over 50: implications for sexual health promotion for older adults. J Sex Med 2010;7(Suppl 5):315–29.
18. Shamu T, Chimbetete C, Egger M, et al. Treatment outcomes in HIV infected patients older than 50 years attending an HIV clinic in Harare, Zimbabwe: a cohort study. PLoS One 2021;16(6):e0253000.
19. Cornell M, Johnson LF, Schomaker M, et al. Age in antiretroviral therapy programmes in South Africa: a retrospective, multicentre, observational cohort study. Lancet HIV 2015;2(9):e368–75.

20. Guerville FVM, Cognet C, Duffau P, et al, on the behalf of ANRS CO3 Aquitaine/AquiVIH-NA study group. Mechanisms of systemic low-grade inflammation in HIV patients on long-term suppressive antiretroviral therapy: the inflammasome hypothesis. AIDS 2023;37(7):1035–46.
21. Quiros-Roldan E, Magoni M, Raffetti E, et al. The burden of chronic diseases and cost-of-care in subjects with HIV infection in a Health District of Northern Italy over a 12-year period compared to that of the general population. BMC Publ Health 2016;16(1):1146.
22. Meir-Shafrir K, Pollack S. Accelerated aging in HIV patients. Rambam Maimonides Med J 2012;3(4):e0025.
23. Tinetti M, Huang A, Molnar F. The geriatrics 5m's: a new way of communicating what we do. J Am Geriatr Soc 2017;65(9):2115.
24. Wastesson JW, Morin L, Tan ECK, et al. An update on the clinical consequences of polypharmacy in older adults: a narrative review. Expet Opin Drug Saf 2018; 17(12):1185–96.
25. Rankin A, Cadogan CA, Patterson SM, et al. Interventions to improve the appropriate use of polypharmacy for older people. Cochrane Database Syst Rev 2018; 9(9):CD008165.
26. Moore KL, Patel K, Boscardin WJ, et al. Medication burden attributable to chronic co-morbid conditions in the very old and vulnerable. PLoS One 2018;13(4): e0196109.
27. Akgün KM, Krishnan S, Tate J, et al. Delirium among people aging with and without HIV: role of alcohol and Neurocognitively active medications. J Am Geriatr Soc 2023;71(6):1861–72.
28. Sung M, Gordon K, Edelman EJ, et al. Polypharmacy and frailty among persons with HIV. AIDS Care 2020;1–8. https://doi.org/10.1080/09540121.2020.1813872.
29. Womack JA, Murphy TE, Rentsch CT, et al. Polypharmacy, hazardous alcohol and illicit substance use and serious falls among PLWH and uninfected comparators. J Acquir Immune Defic Syndr 2019. https://doi.org/10.1097/qai.0000000000002130.
30. Justice AC, Gordon KS, Skanderson M, et al. Nonantiretroviral polypharmacy and adverse health outcomes among HIV-infected and uninfected individuals. AIDS 2018;32(6):739–49.
31. Justice AC, Gordon KS, Romero J, et al. Polypharmacy-associated risk of hospitalisation among people ageing with and without HIV: an observational study. Lancet Healthy Longev 2021;2(10):e639–50.
32. El Moussaoui M, Lambert I, Maes N, et al. Evolution of drug interactions with antiretroviral medication in people with HIV. Open Forum Infect Dis 2020;7(11): ofaa416.
33. Sangiovanni RJ, Jakeman B, Nasiri M, et al. Short communication: relationship between contraindicated drug-drug interactions and subsequent hospitalizations among patients living with HIV initiating combination antiretroviral therapy. AIDS Res Hum Retrovir 2019;35(5):430–3.
34. Lopez-Centeno B, Badenes-Olmedo C, Mataix-Sanjuan A, et al. Polypharmacy and drug-drug interactions in people living with human immunodeficiency virus in the region of madrid, Spain: a population-based study. Clin Infect Dis 2020; 71(2):353–62.
35. Peyro-Saint-Paul L, Besnier P, Demessine L, et al. Cushing's syndrome due to interaction between ritonavir or cobicistat and corticosteroids: a case-control study in the French Pharmacovigilance Database. J Antimicrob Chemother 2019;74(11):3291–4.

36. Mind Exchange Working G. Assessment, diagnosis, and treatment of HIV-associated neurocognitive disorder: a consensus report of the mind exchange program. Clin Infect Dis 2013;56(7):1004–17.
37. Nasreddine ZS. MoCA test mandatory training and certification: what is the purpose? J Am Geriatr Soc 2020;68(2):444–5.
38. Janssen MA, Bosch M, Koopmans PP, et al. Validity of the montreal cognitive assessment and the HIV dementia scale in the assessment of cognitive impairment in HIV-1 infected patients. J Neurovirol 2015;21(4):383–90.
39. Michels TC, Tiu AY, Graver CJ. Neuropsychological evaluation in primary care. Am Fam Physician 2010;82(5):495–502.
40. Nasreddine ZS, Phillips NA, Bedirian V, et al. The montreal cognitive assessment, MoCA: a brief screening tool for mild cognitive impairment. J Am Geriatr Soc 2005;53(4):695–9.
41. Basic D, Rowland JT, Conforti DA, et al. The validity of the Rowland Universal Dementia Assessment Scale (RUDAS) in a multicultural cohort of community-dwelling older persons with early dementia. Alzheimer Dis Assoc Disord Apr-Jun 2009;23(2):124–9.
42. Storey JE, Rowland JT, Basic D, et al. The rowland universal dementia assessment scale (RUDAS): a multicultural cognitive assessment scale. Int Psychogeriatr 2004;16(1):13–31.
43. Xue QL. The frailty syndrome: definition and natural history. Clin Geriatr Med 2011;27(1):1–15.
44. Rockwood K, Bergman H. FRAILTY: a Report from the 3(rd) joint workshop of IAGG/WHO/SFGG, Athens, January 2012. Can Geriatr J 2012;15(2):31–6.
45. Harris TG, Rabkin M, El-Sadr WM. Achieving the fourth 90: healthy aging for people living with HIV. AIDS 2018;32(12):1563–9.
46. Dent E, Kowal P, Hoogendijk EO. Frailty measurement in research and clinical practice: a review. Eur J Intern Med 2016;31:3–10.
47. Justice AC, Tate JP. Strengths and limitations of the veterans aging cohort study index as a measure of physiologic frailty. AIDS Res Hum Retrovir 2019;35(11–12):1023–33.
48. Piggott DA, Erlandson KM, Yarasheski KE. Frailty in HIV: epidemiology, biology, measurement, interventions, and research needs. Curr HIV AIDS Rep 2016;13(6):340–8.
49. Lorenz DR, Mukerji SS, Misra V, et al. Predictors of transition to frailty in middle-aged and older people with HIV: a prospective cohort study. J Acquir Immune Defic Syndr 2021;88(5):518–27.
50. McMillan JM, Gill MJ, Power C, et al. Comorbidities in older persons with controlled HIV infection: correlations with frailty index subtypes. AIDS Patient Care STDS 2020;34(7):284–94.
51. Sun-Suslow N, Paolillo EW, Morgan EE, et al. Brief report: frailty and HIV disease severity synergistically increase risk of HIV-associated neurocognitive disorders. J Acquir Immune Defic Syndr 2020;84(5):522–6.
52. Chen C, Cao X, Xu J, et al. Comparison of healthspan-related indicators between adults with and without HIV infection aged 18-59 in the United States: a secondary analysis of NAHNES 1999-March 2020. BMC Publ Health 2023;23(1):814.
53. Dent E, Morley JE, Cruz-Jentoft AJ, et al. Physical Frailty: ICFSR international clinical practice guidelines for identIFICATION AND MANAGEment. J Nutr Health Aging 2019;23(9):771–87.
54. Cesari M, Gambassi G, van Kan GA, et al. The frailty phenotype and the frailty index: different instruments for different purposes. Age Ageing 2014;43(1):10–2.

55. Sangarlangkarn A, Appelbaum JS. Comprehensive geriatric assessment in older persons with HIV. Open Forum Infect Dis 2020;7(11):ofaa485.
56. Kehler DS, Milic J, Guaraldi G, et al. Frailty in older people living with HIV: current status and clinical management. BMC Geriatr 2022;22(1):919.
57. Erlandson KM, Piggott DA. Frailty and HIV: moving from characterization to intervention. Curr HIV AIDS Rep 2021;18(3):157–75.
58. Sherrington C, Fairhall NJ, Wallbank GK, et al. Exercise for preventing falls in older people living in the community. Cochrane Database Syst Rev 2019;1(1): CD012424.
59. Erlandson KM, Allshouse AA, Jankowski CM, et al. Risk factors for falls in HIV-infected persons. J Acquir Immune Defic Syndr 2012;61(4):484–9.
60. Charumbira MY, Berner K, Louw QA. Falls in people living with HIV: a scoping review. BMJ Open 2020;10(11):e034872.
61. Vaishya R, Vaish A. Falls in older adults are serious. Indian J Orthop 2020;54(1): 69–74.
62. Drewes J, Ebert J, Langer PC, et al. Comorbidities and psychosocial factors as correlates of self-reported falls in a nationwide sample of community-dwelling people aging with HIV in Germany. BMC Publ Health 2021;21(1):1544.
63. Halloran MO, Boyle C, Kehoe B, et al. Polypharmacy and drug-drug interactions in older and younger people living with HIV: the POPPY study. Antivir Ther 2019; 24(3):193–201.
64. Ahmed M, Mital D, Abubaker NE, et al. Bone health in people living with HIV/AIDS: an update of where we are and potential future strategies. Microorganisms 2023;11(3). https://doi.org/10.3390/microorganisms11030789.
65. McComsey GA, Tebas P, Shane E, et al. Bone disease in HIV infection: a practical review and recommendations for HIV care providers. Clin Infect Dis 2010;51(8): 937–46.
66. Battalora L, Buchacz K, Armon C, et al. Low bone mineral density and risk of incident fracture in HIV-infected adults. Antivir Ther 2016;21(1):45–54.
67. Rodriguez M, Daniels B, Gunawardene S, et al. High frequency of vitamin D deficiency in ambulatory HIV-positive patients. AIDS Res Hum Retrovir 2009; 25(1):9–14.
68. Cosman F, de Beur SJ, LeBoff MS, et al. Clinician's guide to prevention and treatment of osteoporosis. Osteoporos Int 2014;25(10):2359–81.
69. Cosman F, de Beur SJ, LeBoff MS, et al, National Osteoporosis Foundation. Clinician's guide to prevention and treatment of osteoporosis. Osteoporos Int 2014;25(10):2359–81.
70. Whetten K, Reif S, Whetten R, et al. Trauma, mental health, distrust, and stigma among HIV-positive persons: implications for effective care. Psychosom Med 2008;70(5):531–8.
71. Brown MJ, Adeagbo O. HIV and aging: double stigma. Curr Epidemiol Rep 2021; 8(2):72–8.
72. Sok P, Gardner S, Bekele T, et al. Unmet basic needs negatively affect health-related quality of life in people aging with HIV: results from the Positive Spaces, Healthy Places study. BMC Publ Health 2018;18(1):644.
73. Umberson D, Montez JK. Social relationships and health: a flashpoint for health policy. J Health Soc Behav 2010;51(Suppl):S54–66.
74. Greene M, Hessol NA, Perissinotto C, et al. Loneliness in older adults living with HIV. AIDS Behav 2018;22(5):1475–84.
75. Hiedemann B, Brodoff L. Increased risks of needing long-term care among older adults living with same-sex partners. Am J Publ Health 2013;103(8):e27–33.

76. Deren S, Cortes T, Dickson VV, et al. Substance use among older people living with HIV: challenges for health care providers. Front Public Health 2019;7:94.
77. Kalokhe AS, Riddick C, Piper K, et al. Integrating program-tailored universal trauma screening into HIV care: an evidence-based participatory approach. AIDS Care 2020;32(2):209–16.
78. Mattson M, Lipari RN, Hays C, et al. A day in the life of older adults: substance use facts. The CBHSQ Report 2013;1–7.
79. Bradley KA, McDonell MB, Bush K, et al. The AUDIT alcohol consumption questions: reliability, validity, and responsiveness to change in older male primary care patients. Alcohol Clin Exp Res 1998;22(8):1842–9.
80. Crane HM, McCaul ME, Chander G, et al. Prevalence and factors associated with hazardous alcohol use among persons living with HIV across the us in the current era of antiretroviral treatment. AIDS Behav 2017;21(7):1914–25.
81. Montgomery L, Bagot K, Brown JL, et al. The association between marijuana use and HIV continuum of care outcomes: a systematic review. Curr HIV AIDS Rep 2019;16(1):17–28.
82. Manuzak JA, Granche J, Tassiopoulos K, et al. Cannabis use is associated with decreased antiretroviral therapy adherence among older adults with HIV. Open Forum Infect Dis 2023;10(1):ofac699.
83. Costiniuk CT, Jenabian MA. Cannabinoids and inflammation: implications for people living with HIV. AIDS 2019;33(15):2273–88.
84. Raymond HF, Chen YH, Ick T, et al. A new trend in the HIV epidemic among men who have sex with men, San Francisco, 2004-2011. J Acquir Immune Defic Syndr 2013;62(5):584–9.
85. Olem D, Earle M, Gomez W, et al. Finding sunshine on a cloudy day: a positive affect intervention for co-occurring methamphetamine use and HIV. Cognit Behav Pract 2022;29(2):267–79.

Mental Health for LGBTQIA+ Older Adults

Rohin A. Aggarwal, MD, MPH[a,*], Cynthia D. Fields, MD[b], Maria H. van Zuilen, PhD[c]

KEYWORDS

• LGBTQIA+ • Older adults • Mental health • Minority stress • Trauma-informed care

KEY POINTS

- Older adults who identify as LGBTQIA+ experience stigma and discrimination that is long-standing and extends to a more oppressive historical era for the community. The minority stress and allostatic load models link these experiences with negative mental and physical health outcomes.
- Because of unique risk factors, LGBTQIA+ older adults experience increased rates of depression, anxiety, and substance use compared with cisgender heterosexual older adults. They also have higher rates of post-traumatic stress disorder, which necessitates the use of a trauma-informed approach to care.
- With smaller and often nontraditional support networks, LGBTQIA+ older adults experience social isolation and loneliness to a higher degree than the general population. This is just one of risk factor for the development of memory loss and cognitive decline.
- Resilience is a positive outcome of the adversity faced by LGBTQIA+ older adults that can prepare individuals for the aging process and lead to improved physical and mental health outcomes.

INTRODUCTION

Older adults in the Lesbian, Gay, Bisexual, Transgender, Queer/Questioning, Intersex, Asexual/Agender (LGBTQIA)+ community share a history of trauma and resilience that continues to impact mental health outcomes and perpetuate disparities compared with their cisgender heterosexual counterparts. Social acceptance in the community and health care spaces has increased, but this does not eliminate the effects of structural barriers and trauma that last throughout the lifespan. The collective

[a] Department of Medicine, Johns Hopkins University School of Medicine, 1800 Orleans Street, Baltimore, MD 21287, USA; [b] Department of Psychiatry and Behavioral Sciences, Johns Hopkins University School of Medicine, 600 North Wolfe Street, Meyer 235, Baltimore, MD 21287, USA; [c] Department of Medical Education, University of Miami Miller School of Medicine (R53), 1600 NW 19th Avenue, Miami, FL 33136, USA

* Corresponding author.

E-mail address: raggarw3@jhmi.edu

Clin Geriatr Med 40 (2024) 299–308

https://doi.org/10.1016/j.cger.2023.10.003

geriatric.theclinics.com

0749-0690/24/

historical and contemporary experiences of LGBTQIA+ older adults in the United States are important context for mental health outcomes that affect this community even today. Oppressive policies have existed throughout the lifespan of older adults, from the McCarthy era in the 1950s to "Don't Ask, Don't Tell" in the 1990s to the increase in statewide bans of gender-affirming care in 2023.[1,2] LGBTQIA+ older adults have also demonstrated strength to advocate for a more equitable environment, beginning with the Stonewall Uprising of 1969, calling for focused attention on destigmatizing and treating Human Immunodeficiency Virus/Acquired Immunodeficiency Syndrome (HIV/AIDS), and rejecting "homosexuality" and "gender identity disorder" as pathologic conditions included in the Diagnostic and Statistical Manual of Mental Disorders.[1–3] This article focuses on the unique factors that impact mental health for LGBTQIA+ older adults and illustrates how health care providers can deliver culturally competent, trauma-informed, and holistic care to this population.

MINORITY STRESS AND ALLOSTATIC LOAD

Mental health concerns among LGBTQIA+ individuals must be considered under the minority stress model, a framework that has been used as the primary explanation for health disparities in this population.[4,5] The minority stress model describes the creation of a hostile and stressful social environment that ultimately leads to increased rates and severity of mental health issues for those affected by stigma, prejudice, and discrimination. Minority stress related to the experience of LGBTQIA+ individuals is categorized into distal, or external, stressors (ie, objective prejudiced or discriminatory events) and proximal, or internal, stressors (ie, nonconsensual disclosure or concealment of identities, anticipation of discrimination, internalized homophobia or transphobia).[4,6] The allostatic load model has additionally been adopted to conceptualize pathophysiological effects of cumulative "wear and tear" due to chronic stressors.[5,7–9] Allostatic load has been linked to the hypothalamic–pituitary–adrenal axis and multiple biomarkers (such as cortisol), which ultimately leads to dysregulation of the cardiovascular, gastrointestinal, endocrine, and immune systems.[9,10]

Both the minority stress and allostatic load models can help clinicians understand the link between experiences of LGBTQIA+ older adults and their individual and collective health. Many LGBTQIA+ older adults have also had negative experiences with providers in clinical spaces, resulting in collective distrust of the health care system. These cumulative stressors ultimately lead to the increased rates of chronic disease, including mental health conditions that could have been prevented or treated earlier.[11] Transgender and gender diverse (TGD) individuals have been at the forefront of civil rights efforts and have unique stressors related to oppressive legislation that continues to negatively impact equitable access to gender-affirming care.[12] A 2022 study noted higher allostatic load measured with biomarkers among transmasculine participants who lived in perceptibly less progressive geopolitical climates with lower sociodemographic advantage.[13] In an effort to reduce distrust and encourage earlier interactions with the health care system, clinicians should increase their own awareness and knowledge of seminal events (ie, the Stonewall riots), contemporary geopolitical changes, and the daily experiences of stigma that impact the LGBTQIA+ community.[14]

IDENTITY DISCLOSURE AND SELF-ACCEPTANCE

"Coming out" encompasses both identity disclosure and the journey of one's acceptance of their own identity.[14,15] For every individual, coming out is a unique and iterative process driven by multiple factors, such as the surrounding geopolitical and cultural environment.[15,16] For many LGBTQIA+ older adults, the process can take decades and is coupled with years of identity concealment due to fear of discrimination.[17] Identity disclosure can be a complex and sometimes traumatic experience for LGBTQIA+ older adults.[17,18] On an individual level, negative prior experiences with disclosure in the setting of a homophobic, biphobic, or transphobic environment affect one's willingness to come out later in life.[14] The internalization of stigma related to sexual and gender minority identities, otherwise known as internalized homophobia or transphobia, involves a person's negative feelings about their own identity as influenced by the society around them.[19] Understanding the historical stigma against LGBTQIA+ older adults is essential when providing affirming, trauma-informed care (TIC), and the decision to disclose identity in the health care setting should rest with the patient.[20] Terminology surrounding sexual and gender minorities is evolving, and the patient should be in full control of how they describe and label their own identity rather than having one prescribed to them by a provider.[20,21] For example, although the term "queer" has been reclaimed by the community, it can be triggering or distressing to LGBTQIA+ older adults who may have previously been addressed as "queer" in a derogatory manner.[21]

SOCIAL ISOLATION AND LONELINESS

Social isolation is defined as having a low quantity and quality of contact with others, whereas loneliness is the feeling of isolation regardless of the objective social network size.[22] Both have generally been associated with a variety of physical and psychosocial issues for older adults, including increased depression, falls, functional decline, hospital admissions, and even mortality.[22,23] LGBTQIA+ older adults have higher rates of social isolation and loneliness than the general older adult population for multiple reasons due to perceived and anticipated discrimination.[12,14,23] According to a survey conducted by the American Association of Retired Persons, most LGBTQIA+ older adults are concerned about the level of support from family and friends as they age.[22] Contrary to typical family and social networks found among many cisgender heterosexual individuals, those of LGBTQIA+ older adults are often nontraditional due to rejection by the biological or legal family with the subsequent formation of "chosen families."[14,23] LGBTQIA+ older adults are also less likely to have intergenerational wealth or children who can provide social, financial, and caregiver support, which can lead to significant physical and mental health disparities.[12,22,24] These factors are barriers to continued independence in the community and result in higher levels of vulnerability within environments that could be discriminatory, such as elder care settings (ie, long-term facilities, nursing homes, assisted living).[25] One qualitative study in particular interviewed TGD individuals and found several common themes related to aging, including perceived lack of agency, vulnerability to financial stressors, isolation exacerbated by gender identity, and fear of mistreatment under the care of others.[12] LGBTQIA+ older adults in elder care settings—especially those who are more dependent by the way of cognitive impairment or mobility issues—may have negative experiences, from blatant harassment to refusal by staff to provide care.[18,23,26,27] It has been shown that LGBTQIA+ older adults who receive care and live in an environment that is affirming of their identities experience fewer negative mental health consequences.[18,26] Many LGBTQIA+ older adults prioritize "aging in place," or living at home in familiar communities for as long as possible.[25] Providers can support LGBTQIA+ older adults in achieving this goal by focusing on preservation of independence, having earlier goals-of-care conversations, and preparing legal documents (ie, advance directives, living will, and powers of attorney).[24,28]

DEPRESSION AND ANXIETY

Depression and anxiety disproportionately affect LGBTQIA+ older adults in the United States as a direct result of increased rates of social isolation and loneliness.[29] Depression also increases among those with lower social network sizes or those who live alone, which tends to be more prevalent among the LGBTQIA+ population.[29,30] Of note, the mental health effects of quarantining during the COVID-19 pandemic were found to be higher for LGBTQIA+ older adults due to worsening of social isolation beyond baseline.[31,32] Other risk factors include bereavement, cognitive impairment, and increased prevalence of chronic disease among older adults.[33] Depression and anxiety have been associated with negative physical health impacts, including obesity, cardiovascular disease, obstructive pulmonary disease, and increased hospitalization, morbidity, and mortality related to these conditions.[33–35] Unique to the LGBTQIA+ population is the significant impact of HIV, especially among an aging population whose lived experience was affected by the epidemic. Depression and anxiety have been linked to increased sexual risk behavior among men who have sex with men (MSM) and, for MSM who live with HIV, higher viral loads and decreased antiretroviral therapy adherence.[30,36,37] Physical ability or activity is shown to be protective against psychological distress; however, many older adults do not benefit from this protective factor given that mobility declines with aging.[38] Another protective mechanism is "mastery," or the sense of control that an individual feels that they have over various aspects of their lives and events that occur around them.[38] In elder care settings, one's sense of control may be compromised, potentially leading to identity concealment and increased risk of depression and anxiety.[18,31] Increased mastery has been associated with lower rates of depression and anxiety, as well as an improvement in quality of life as perceived by LGBTQIA+ older adults.[25,38]

POST-TRAUMATIC STRESS DISORDER AND TRAUMA-INFORMED CARE

The experience of trauma is one of shared identity for LGBTQIA+ older adults who have lived during eras when same-sex sexual and gender-nonconforming behaviors and identities were considered morally, pathologically, and legally divergent from accepted social norms.[39] Trauma has known psychological consequences, leading to increased rates of depression, anxiety, post-traumatic stress disorder (PTSD), substance use, and health risk behaviors.[39] PTSD is linked not only to life-threatening or physically violent events but can also encompass effects from identity concealment that result in self-afflicted shame, internalized homo/transphobia, and social avoidance.[39,40] The health care system is similarly responsible for inflicting traumatic experiences rooted in blatant discrimination or microaggressions.[41] A revealing report published in 2010 by Lambda Legal showed that about 56% of LGB respondents and 70% of TGD respondents reported at least one of the following: being refused needed care, being blamed for their health status, or abusive language or physical abuse from health care providers.[41,42] For LGBTQIA+ older adults who also belong to a racial minority group, the rate of negative or traumatic experiences within the health care system is even higher compared with non-Hispanic white members of the community.[43] In addition, LGBTQIA+ older adults are at an increased risk of experiencing domestic elder abuse, neglect, and exploitation by caregivers due to their sexual orientation or gender identity.[44] It should be noted that many of these incidents go unreported due to understandable distrust in authorities, especially given historically afflicted trauma on the community by law enforcement and the judicial system.[39,44]

Given that health disparities are exacerbated by individual and collective trauma, it is important to adopt a trauma-informed approach when caring for LGBTQIA+ older adults.[41,45] TIC is a comprehensive, culturally competent framework that emphasizes trust-building, elimination of power dynamics, and resistance of re-traumatization by providers.[45] TIC can encompass how a clinician approaches the physical examination, discusses treatment options, or recognizes signs and symptoms of trauma during patient–provider interactions.[41,44,45] A significant component of TIC for LGBTQIA+ older adults is a thorough understanding of both the historical and contemporary sociopolitical environments that affect mental health.[44,45] In addition, TIC requires addressing one's own implicit or unconscious biases and how that may affect the ability to equitably care for LGBTQIA+ older adults.[41] Recognizing one's own discomfort and reactivity to unfamiliar clinical situations is paramount to counteracting the risk of contributing to a patient's trauma burden.[41,43] Information surrounding best practices in TIC with specific ways to counteract implicit bias have been well-described in other sources.[39,41,45,46]

SUBSTANCE USE

Substance use among LGBTQIA+ older adults is complex and driven by many factors, including minority stress, environmental exposures, and social norms.[44] In particular, alcohol and tobacco use are more prevalent among the community and under the minority stress model have been labeled as a coping behavior when stressors are outside one's control.[19,32] Historically, the sociopolitical environment, legal discrimination, and victimization of the community by police led to the development of an underground bar and nightclub scene where alcohol, tobacco, and other substances were readily available.[44,47] On a more contemporary note, the prevalence of substance use increased among LGBTQIA+ older adults during the COVID-19 pandemic.[32] It is important to recognize that substance use prevalence differs between populations within the LGBTQIA+ community. Although research specific to TGD older adults and rates of substance use is rather limited, one study found higher rates of chronic pain (a risk factor for opioid misuse) among TGD Medicare recipients compared with cisgender individuals.[40,48] Another study showed that completion of successful gender affirmation surgery correlates with decreased tobacco use among TGD patients.[49] Regarding alcohol use among TGD individuals, minimal evidence exists to determine a threshold for hazardous alcohol use, given that the National Institute on Alcohol Abuse and Alcoholism uses gendered cutoffs based on data from cisgender individuals.[40] Efforts to address substance use among the LGBTQIA+ community often target younger populations, and those that address substance use for the older adult population do not have components specific to LGBTQIA+ older adults.[44,47] As substance use among older adults is generally underreported, screening for substance use among LGBTQIA+ older adults is of particular importance in primary care settings.

MEMORY AND COGNITIVE IMPAIRMENT

LGBTQIA+ older adults have a distinct combination of risk factors (ie, minority stress) that can lead to memory loss and cognitive impairment.[17,47,50] Historical, institutional, and societal discrimination have been linked to higher prevalence of physical and psychosocial health issues in LGBTQIA+ older adults, which are considered modifiable risk factors for cognitive impairment and dementia.[6,51–53] For LGBTQIA+ older adults who also identify as a racial or ethnic minority, the prevalence of subjective cognitive decline is even higher.[51,54] With memory loss and cognitive impairment, there are concerns for loss of agency or sense of control, which may affect LGBTQIA+ older adults by the way of retraumatization.[51,54] Especially among TGD older adults, there is a fear of loss of control over a personal narrative, which may be altered by family members who are not supportive of their transition or affirming of their gender identity.[12,55] To promote affirming care to LGBTQIA+ older adults, it is crucial that providers plan in advance with patients to complete legal documentation, such as advance directives, funeral directives, and living wills. The goal is to preserve the legal authority and autonomy for LGBTQIA+ older adults and their partners should the patient be incapacitated as a result of cognitive decline or severe illness.[54]

RESILIENCE AND COMMUNITY

It is important to recognize that despite the mental health disparities described in this article, LGBTQIA+ older adults have overcome significant barriers and stressors by the way of forming strong communities and exhibiting resilience.[56,57] Resilience is defined as a process and outcome of successfully adapting to difficult or challenging life experiences, especially through mental, emotional, and behavioral flexibility and adjustment to external and internal demands.[56,58] In an effort to reduce pathologizing of sexual orientation and gender diversity, the minority resilience hypothesis argues that stigma and discrimination do not only negatively impact individuals but also foster adaptation in the face of adversity.[6,40] Although negative health outcomes as a result of minority stress and allostatic load are very real, having experienced these unique stressors may better position LGBTQIA+ older adults to cope with the challenges of aging and lead to better mental health outcomes.[56,57,59] One important example is the coming out process, which eventually results in the development of authenticity, growth in both social and personal identity, improvement in mental health, and involvement in advocacy efforts.[56,60] Other protective factors that contribute to resilience include social support and affirmation, creating role model and mentee relationships, and community building.[40,56]

Community building is central to LGBTQIA+ culture and has created enormous support networks for LGBTQIA+ older adults historically.[56,59] Many LGBTQIA+ older adults have, in response to rejection from their biological families, formed chosen families that create a positive and affirming atmosphere for identity exploration and expression.[44] Clinicians in conjunction with social work and case management staff should be aware of and refer patients to communities and organizations that serve LGBTQIA+ older adults.[44,56] Resources that target and improve health outcomes for older adults are not always inclusive of the unique needs of LGBTQIA+ older adults, and providers should advocate for and contribute to the development of equitable programs and policies that support the LGBTQIA+ community.[56,61]

CLINICS CARE POINTS

- Providers have a responsibility to understand the collective historical and modern sources of stress that negatively impact LGBTQIA+ communities.
- LGBTQIA+ older adults are at higher risk of depression, anxiety, social isolation, post-traumatic stress disorder, substance use disorders, and cognitive impairment due to cumulative minority stress and allostatic load.
- Support networks among LGBTQIA+ older adults are often nontraditional. Providers should have early discussions with patients about preferences for medical decision-making and legal documentation to preserve autonomy and prevent vulnerability.
- Few equitable programs for older adults exist that also support the unique needs of LGBTQIA+ older adults and should be advocated for by the medical community.

- Providers should facilitate the training of all staff members on trauma-informed practices and delivering affirming care to LGBTQIA+ older adults in clinical and elder care settings.
- Resilience and strong community building are positive outcomes of adversity faced by LGBTQIA+ older adults and are protective for mental and physical health throughout the aging process.

DISCLOSURE

The authors have nothing to disclose.

REFERENCES

1. Goldsen KF. Shifting social context in the lives of LGBTQ older adults. In: Hudson RB, editor. Public Policy Aging Rep 2018;28(1):24–8. https://doi.org/10.1093/ppar/pry003.
2. Shapiro S, Powell T. Medical Intervention and LGBT people: a brief history. In: Eckstrand KL, Potter J, editors. Trauma, resilience, and health promotion in LGBT patients: what every healthcare provider should know. Springer International Publishing; 2017. p. 15–23. https://doi.org/10.1007/978-3-319-54509-7_2.
3. Drescher J. Out of DSM: depathologizing homosexuality. Behav Sci Basel Switz 2015;5(4):565–75.
4. Flentje A, Heck NC, Brennan JM, et al. The relationship between minority stress and biological outcomes: a systematic review. J Behav Med 2020;43(5):673–94.
5. Desjardins G, Caceres BA, Juster RP. Sexual minority health and allostatic load in the National Health and Nutrition Examination Survey: a systematic scoping review with intersectional implications. Psychoneuroendocrinology 2022;145:105916.
6. Meyer IH. Prejudice, social stress, and mental health in lesbian, gay, and bisexual populations: conceptual issues and research evidence. Psychol Bull 2003;129(5):674–97.
7. McEwen BS, Stellar E. Stress and the individual. Mechanisms leading to disease. Arch Intern Med 1993;153(18):2093–101.
8. McEwen BS. Stress, adaptation, and disease. Allostasis and allostatic load. Ann N Y Acad Sci 1998;840:33–44.
9. Guidi J, Lucente M, Sonino N, et al. Allostatic load and its impact on health: a systematic review. Psychother Psychosom 2021;90(1):11–27.
10. Seeman TE, McEwen BS, Rowe JW, et al. Allostatic load as a marker of cumulative biological risk: MacArthur studies of successful aging. Proc Natl Acad Sci U S A 2001;98(8):4770–5.
11. Hoy-Ellis CP, Ator M, Kerr C, et al. Innovative approaches address aging and mental health needs in LGBTQ communities. Published online 2017.
12. Adan M, Scribani M, Tallman N, et al. Worry and wisdom: a qualitative study of transgender elders' perspectives on aging. Transgender Health 2021;6(6):332–42.
13. DuBois LZ, Juster RP. Lived experience and allostatic load among transmasculine people living in the United States. Psychoneuroendocrinology 2022;143:105849.
14. Streed CG, Adams M, Terndrup C, et al. Adult primary care. In: Lehman JR, Diaz K, Ng H, et al, editors. The equal curriculum. Springer International Publishing; 2020. p. 107–29. https://doi.org/10.1007/978-3-030-24025-7_7.

15. Walker M, McGrath M. Gender identity emergence and affirmation in adults. In: Keuroghlian AS, Potter J, Reisner SL, editors. Transgender and gender diverse health care: the fenway guide. McGraw Hill; 2022. Available at: accessmedicine.mhmedical.com/content.aspx?aid=1184175985. Accessed August 14, 2023.
16. Leung E. Thematic analysis of my "coming out" experiences through an intersectional lens: an autoethnographic study. Front Psychol 2021;12:654946.
17. Fredriksen-Goldsen KI, Kim HJ, Shiu C, et al. Successful aging among LGBT older adults: physical and mental health-related quality of life by age group. Gerontol 2015;55(1):154–68.
18. Miller LR. Queer aging: older lesbian, gay, and bisexual adults' visions of late life. Innov Aging 2023;7(3):igad021.
19. Institute of Medicine (US), Committee on lesbian, gay, bisexual, and transgender health issues and research gaps and opportunities. The health of lesbian, gay, bisexual, and transgender people: building a foundation for better understanding. National Academies Press (US); 2011. Available at: http://www.ncbi.nlm.nih.gov/books/NBK64806/. Accessed August 14, 2023.
20. Heredia D, Pankey TL, Gonzalez CA. LGBTQ-affirmative behavioral health services in primary care. Prim Care 2021;48(2):243–57.
21. Worthen MGF. Queer identities in the 21st century: reclamation and stigma. Curr Opin Psychol 2023;49:101512.
22. Freedman A, Nicolle J. Social isolation and loneliness: the new geriatric giants: approach for primary care. Can Fam Physician Med Fam Can 2020;66(3):176–82.
23. Kuyper L, Fokkema T. Loneliness among older lesbian, gay, and bisexual adults: the role of minority stress. Arch Sex Behav 2010;39(5):1171–80.
24. Jackson Levin N, Kattari SK, Piellusch EK, et al. "We just take care of each other": navigating 'chosen family' in the context of health, illness, and the mutual provision of care amongst queer and transgender young adults. Int J Environ Res Public Health 2020;17(19):7346.
25. Boggs JM, Dickman Portz J, King DK, et al. Perspectives of LGBTQ older adults on aging in place: a qualitative Investigation. J Homosex 2017;64(11):1539–60.
26. Neville S, Henrickson M. "Lavender retirement": a questionnaire survey of lesbian, gay and bisexual people's accommodation plans for old age. Int J Nurs Pract 2010;16(6):586–94.
27. McGovern J, Brown D, Gasparro V. Lessons learned from an LGBTQ senior center: a Bronx tale. J Gerontol Soc Work 2016;59(7–8):496–511.
28. Preston R. Quality of life among LGBTQ older adults in the United States: a systematic review. J Am Psychiatr Nurses Assoc 2022. https://doi.org/10.1177/10783903221127697. 107839032211276.
29. Steinman L, Parrish A, Mayotte C, et al. Increasing social connectedness for underserved older adults living with depression: a pre-post evaluation of PEARLS. Am J Geriatr Psychiatry 2021;29(8):828–42.
30. Henderson ER, Egan JE, Haberlen SA, et al. Does social support predict depressive symptoms? A longitudinal study of midlife and older men who have sex with men from the multicenter AIDS cohort study. Ann LGBTQ Public Popul Health 2021;2(2):142–60.
31. Chen JH. Disparities in mental health and well-being between heterosexual and sexual minority older adults during the COVID-19 pandemic. J Aging Health 2022;34(6–8):939–50.
32. Akré ER, Anderson A, Stojanovski K, et al. Depression, anxiety, and alcohol use among LGBTQ+ people during the COVID-19 pandemic. Am J Public Health 2021;111(9):1610–9.

33. Maier A, Riedel-Heller SG, Pabst A, et al. Risk factors and protective factors of depression in older people 65+. A systematic review. PLoS One 2021;16(5): e0251326.
34. Connolly MJ, Yohannes AM. The impact of depression in older patients with chronic obstructive pulmonary disease and asthma. Maturitas 2016;92:9–14.
35. Zhang Y, Chen Y, Ma L. Depression and cardiovascular disease in elderly: current understanding. J Clin Neurosci 2018;47:1–5.
36. Stall R, Mills TC, Williamson J, et al. Association of co-occurring psychosocial health problems and increased vulnerability to HIV/AIDS among urban men who have sex with men. Am J Public Health 2003;93(6):939–42.
37. Friedman MR, Coulter RWS, Silvestre AJ, et al. Someone to count on: social support as an effect modifier of viral load suppression in a prospective cohort study. AIDS Care 2017;29(4):469–80.
38. Fredriksen Goldsen K, Kim HJ, Jung H, et al. The evolution of aging with pride—national health, aging, and sexuality/gender study: illuminating the iridescent life course of LGBTQ adults aged 80 years and older in the United States. Int J Aging Hum Dev 2019;88(4):380–404.
39. Alessi EJ, Martin JI. Intersection of trauma and identity. In: Eckstrand KL, Potter J, editors. Trauma, resilience, and health promotion in LGBT patients: what every healthcare provider should know. Springer International Publishing; 2017. p. 3–14. https://doi.org/10.1007/978-3-319-54509-7_1.
40. Henin A, Darsney C, Vaz De Souza F, et al. Behavioral health considerations for transgender and gender diverse people. In: Keuroghlian AS, Potter J, Reisner SL, editors. Transgender and gender diverse health care: the fenway guide. McGraw Hill; 2022. Available at: accessmedicine.mhmedical.com/content.aspx?aid=1184176055. Accessed September 5, 2023.
41. Poteat TC, Singh AA. Conceptualizing trauma in clinical settings: Iatrogenic harm and bias. In: Eckstrand KL, Potter J, editors. Trauma, resilience, and health promotion in LGBT patients: what every healthcare provider should know. Springer International Publishing; 2017. p. 25–33. https://doi.org/10.1007/978-3-319-54509-7_3.
42. Lambda Legal. When health care isn't caring: Lambda legal's survey of discrimination against LGBT people and people living with HIV. Lambda Legal; 2010. Available at: https://legacy.lambdalegal.org/sites/default/files/publications/downloads/whcic-report_when-health-care-isnt-caring.pdf.
43. Chen J, McLaren H, Jones M, et al. The aging experiences of LGBTQ ethnic minority older adults: a systematic review. In: Heyn PC, editor. Gerontol 2022;62(3): e162–77. https://doi.org/10.1093/geront/gnaa134.
44. Hoy-Ellis CP. Older adults. In: Eckstrand KL, Potter J, editors. Trauma, resilience, and health promotion in lgbt patients: what every healthcare provider should know. Springer International Publishing; 2017. p. 89–101. https://doi.org/10.1007/978-3-319-54509-7_8.
45. Sciolla AF. An overview of trauma-informed care. In: Eckstrand KL, Potter J, editors. Trauma, resilience, and health promotion in LGBT patients: what every healthcare provider should know. Springer International Publishing; 2017. p. 165–81. https://doi.org/10.1007/978-3-319-54509-7_14.
46. Levenson JS, Craig SL, Austin A. Trauma-informed and affirmative mental health practices with LGBTQ+ clients. Psychol Serv 2023;20(Suppl 1):134–44.
47. Fredriksen-Goldsen KI, Kim HJ, Barkan SE, et al. Health disparities among lesbian, gay, and bisexual older adults: results from a population-based study. Am J Public Health 2013;103(10):1802–9.

48. Dragon CN, Guerino P, Ewald E, et al. Transgender Medicare beneficiaries and chronic conditions: exploring fee-for-service claims data. LGBT Health 2017; 4(6):404–11.
49. Almazan AN, Keuroghlian AS. Association between gender-affirming surgeries and mental health outcomes. JAMA Surg 2021;156(7):611–8.
50. Juster RP, McEwen BS, Lupien SJ. Allostatic load biomarkers of chronic stress and impact on health and cognition. Psychophysiological Biomark Health 2010; 35(1):2–16.
51. Flatt JD, Johnson JK, Karpiak SE, et al. Correlates of subjective cognitive decline in lesbian, gay, bisexual, and transgender older adults. J Alzheimers Dis JAD 2018;64(1):91–102.
52. Fredriksen-Goldsen KI, Kim HJ, Barkan SE. Disability among lesbian, gay, and bisexual adults: disparities in prevalence and risk. Am J Public Health 2012; 102(1):e16–21.
53. Kim HJ, Fredriksen-Goldsen K, Jung HH. Determinants of physical functioning and health-related quality of life among sexual and gender minority older adults with cognitive impairment. J Aging Health 2023;35(1–2):138–50.
54. Fredriksen-Goldsen KI, Jen S, Bryan AEB, et al. Cognitive impairment, Alzheimer's disease, and other dementias in the lives of lesbian, gay, bisexual and transgender (LGBT) older adults and their caregivers: needs and competencies. J Appl Gerontol Off J South Gerontol Soc 2018;37(5):545–69.
55. Lambrou NH, Gleason CE, Obedin-Maliver J, et al. Subjective cognitive decline associated with discrimination in medical settings among transgender and nonbinary older adults. Int J Environ Res Public Health 2022;19(15):9168.
56. Smith NG. Resilience across the life span: adulthood. In: Eckstrand KL, Potter J, editors. Trauma, resilience, and health promotion in LGBT patients: what every healthcare provider should know. Springer International Publishing; 2017. p. 75–88. https://doi.org/10.1007/978-3-319-54509-7_7.
57. Fredriksen-Goldsen KI, Kim HJ, Bryan AEB, et al. The cascading effects of marginalization and pathways of resilience in attaining good health among LGBT older adults. Gerontol 2017;57(suppl 1):S72–83.
58. Southwick SM, Bonanno GA, Masten AS, et al. Resilience definitions, theory, and challenges: interdisciplinary perspectives. Eur J Psychotraumatology 2014;5. https://doi.org/10.3402/ejpt.v5.25338.
59. Yu H, Fan L, Gilliland AJ. Disparities and resilience: analyzing online Health information provision, behaviors and needs of LBGTQ + elders during COVID-19. BMC Publ Health 2022;22(1):2338.
60. Vaughan MD, Waehler CA. Coming out growth: conceptualizing and measuring stress-related growth associated with coming out to others as a sexual minority. J Adult Dev 2010;17(2):94–109.
61. Stinchcombe A, Kortes-Miller K, Wilson K. "We are resilient, we made it to this point": a study of the lived experiences of older LGBTQ2S+ Canadians. J Appl Gerontol 2021;40(11):1533–41.

Psychosocial and Financial Issues Affecting LGBTQ+ Older Adults

Vinita Gidvani Shastri, MD[a,*], Erica Joy Erney, BSW, MSW, LCSW[b]

KEYWORDS

• Isolation • Financial security • Housing • Advance care planning • Long-term care • Caregiving • LGBTQIA+ • Older adult • LGBTQ+

KEY POINTS

- Social connections, financial security, advance care documentation completion, and availability of inclusive long-term care are the cornerstones of psychosocial needs of LGBTQ+ older adults.
- Systemic discrimination reflected in the law, cultural norms, and heteronormative/cisgender practices have limited access to health care and social support systems that would enable LGBTQ+ older adults to age in place.
- Financial insecurity in this population may stem from lower income, lack of savings for retirement, limited availability of safe and affordable housing, and limitations of eligibility for health insurance based on marital status.
- LGBTQ+ older adults are often less prepared for the cost of additional care and more resistant to accessing social support services for fear of discrimination.
- Completion of advance care planning documents ensures that dignity is maintained at the end of life and that assets are protected and distributed in a manner consistent with LGBTQ+ older adults' wishes.

INTRODUCTION

Isolation, financial insecurity, incomplete advance care planning, and need for long-term care are universal concerns of older adults. These psychosocial challenges are further magnified in gender and sexual minorities who have experienced the accumulated effects of systemic discrimination throughout their lifetimes. LGBTQ+ older adults are disproportionately more likely to live alone and experience financial poverty and social isolation stemming from decades of living in the margins of a society that

[a] GRECC, VA Palo Alto Health Care System, Stanford School of Medicine, 3801 Miranda Avenue (182b), Palo Alto, CA 94304, USA; [b] The Permanente Medical Group, Kaiser Permanente Santa Clara Medical Center, 710 Lawrence Expressway, Dept 440 (MOB), Santa Clara, CA 95051, USA
* Corresponding author.
E-mail addresses: gidvaniv@stanford.edu; Vinita.Shastri@va.gov

Clin Geriatr Med 40 (2024) 309–320
https://doi.org/10.1016/j.cger.2023.10.004 geriatric.theclinics.com
0749-0690/24/

has not accepted their identity. This marginalization is reflected systemically in the law, cultural norms, and heteronormative and cisgender practices. LGBTQ+ older adults have been concealing their sexual and gender identity from health care providers and social workers as a method to survive. Aging and its associated functional decline may leave an LGBTQ+ older adult feeling vulnerable to exposure of an identity that they have kept tightly concealed or push them back into the closet after being out for years. LGBTQ+ older adults experiencing cognitive impairment is an especially defenseless population due to their lack of social connection and potential lack of financial resources and advance care planning. This article explores what is currently known about the nuanced financial and psychosocial challenges that LGBTQ+ older adults face (**Fig. 1**).

CLINICAL VIGNETTE (CASE STUDY/PRESENTATION)

It is the year 2012. Yvette is an 82-year-old White who identifies as a transgender lesbian. Amy is a 77-year-old Latina who identifies as a lesbian. They both have had a fraught past with their gender and sexual identities and came out later in life after being estranged from their family of origin. Yvette was never married and has no children. Amy was divorced after a short marriage and has one biological child named Elsa. Amy and Elsa are not on speaking terms. Amy moved away from her hometown as the shame and repudiation from her community was too much for her to bear. Yvette and Amy have now been together for 10 years. They live in separate apartments and have continued to work in their neighborhood bakery to make ends meet. They live quiet lives and are happy.

SOCIAL CONNECTION

Yvette starts to show signs of memory loss. She has been unable to manage the cash register at the bakery. Amy has been trying to cover for her mistakes and this is taking a toll. They both have not seen a doctor in years, but Amy decides it is time for Yvette to be evaluated. Yvette undergoes neuropsychological testing and is diagnosed with mild-stage Alzheimer's disease. Amy accompanies Yvette to the appointment, stating that she is Yvette's good friend and driver.

Amy feels lost after hearing Yvette's diagnosis. She is the only person in Yvette's life, and she never expected to take on the role of caregiver—emotionally or financially. The physician gave her a resource for the clinic support group that she attended one time. Amy found that she was the only one in a same-sex relationship and one participant even made a derogatory comment about a hired "lazy lesbian" caregiver that sat around and did nothing.

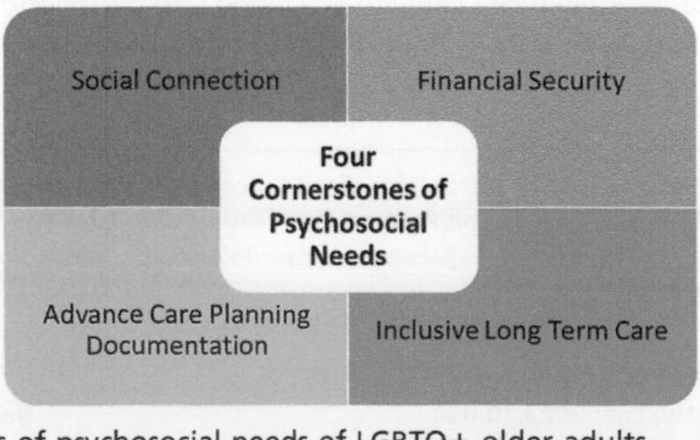

Fig. 1. Cornerstones of psychosocial needs of LGBTQ+ older adults.

The "Invisible Generation," defined as the generation of oldest LGBTQ adults who grew up in a time of no acknowledgment of gender or sexual disparity, has been isolated their entire lives.[1] Research shows that staying connected allows older adults to age well, live longer, and combat cognitive impairment, whereas isolation has the opposite effect.[2,3] LGBTQ+ older adults are twice as likely to be single and live alone and four times less likely to have children than their heterosexual counterparts.[3] Multiple studies indicate that greater than 50% of surveyed LGBTQ+ older adults feel socially isolated.[4,5]

SYSTEMIC DISCRIMINATION

This isolation stems from a lifetime of discrimination where identifying as gay, lesbian, bisexual, transgender, queer, or questioning could have led to arrest, hospitalization for mental illness or lack of employment/harassment in the workplace.[4] LGBTQ+ older adults have spent the majority of their lives living in a society that has not accepted differences in sexual orientation or gender identity as evidenced by the law, policies, and cultural norms. Eighty-two percent of older adults in this community have experienced at least one episode of victimization including verbal threats, harassment, and physical assault with two-thirds experiencing at least three episodes in their lifetime.[4] This discrimination has affected their basic survival needs of employment and housing and led to disparities in physical and mental health.

FAMILIES OF CHOICE

The disparities of sexual and gender minorities are not all the same. Gay men are less likely to be married or have children/grandchildren and more likely to live alone.[5] As function declines and dependency increases with aging, isolation poses a challenge to receiving care. Many LGBTQ+ older adults have experienced difficult and alienating relationships with family, friends, employers, and their communities including health care providers. Many move away from their families of origin to stay in the closet or to distance themselves from the shame and discrimination they have faced.[6] They end up creating "families of choice": a social network composed of found friends and partners, typically of the same generation aging at the same rate, which serve as family.[7]

ACCESS TO SUPPORT SERVICES

Many LGBTQ+ older adults will end up choosing not to access health services including health care, social support, and housing support. If they do, they may choose not to reveal their sexual identity for fear of discrimination and losing the protection of invisibility in which they have been cloaked.[8] As such, LGBTQ+ older adults may not receive the support that they would be eligible for to age in place, to maintain their well-being or access the right level of care should their function decline.

AVOIDANCE OF HEALTH CARE

LGBTQ+ older adults have avoided accessing health care due to concern for discrimination.[6] This concern is even more apparent in transgender older adults. Nearly one in four transgender adults avoid going to the doctor for fear of mistreatment[4]; one in three transgender adults avoid going due to financial concerns leading to isolation not just from peers but from the health care system.[4] The avoidance of care leads to diagnoses at advanced stages of illness with complications that are more difficult to treat.

ISOLATION OF CAREGIVERS

Although one in 13 older LGBTQ+ adults experiences cognitive impairment, being a caregiver for a loved one with this disease has its own imperceptible vulnerability.[9] Many LGBTQ+ adults are thrown into the role of caregiving, with 21% of older LGBTQ+ people providing care to a friend compared with just 6% of non-LGBTQ+ counterparts.[4] Furthermore, they enter this role without engaging in support systems most others take for granted for fear of discrimination and nuanced challenges not addressed in traditional support groups. They often must educate and receive care from non-LGBTQ+ affirming mental health providers. They may also suffer from financial marginalization, which compounds the limited access. Caregivers of LGBTQ+ older adults are more likely to be of the same age as their care recipient and often managing their own health concerns. "Dignity 2022: The Experience of LGBTQ Older Adults" survey found that LGBTQ+ caregivers are emotionally stressed, not getting enough rest, and find it challenging to exercise with a large percentage experiencing their own health problems while balancing work with caregiver responsibilities.[5]

DUAL CAREGIVING ROLE OF LGBTQ+ CAREGIVERS

LGBTQ+ older adults often face the additional challenge of defaulting into the role of caregiver for their aging parents of their family of origin in addition to being the caregiver for their partner or chosen family network. This further compounds the challenge of being able to care for one's own physical, emotional, social, and spiritual well-being.[6]

FINANCIAL SECURITY

Yvette is forced to retire from the bakery. Amy continues to work long hours to save for what she heard from her support group will be a very expensive journey. Neither of them has been able to save much for retirement. They decide to sell Yvette's apartment and look for a lower cost apartment to move in together. However, Amy is worried about leaving Yvette at home alone while she is at work due to safety concerns. They hire a realtor who ends up canceling the majority of their apartment viewings last minute and they are questioned about the nature of their relationship by the mortgage lender at the bank. Amy decides to install a video camera at home to watch Yvette instead of applying for social support or looking into a home care agency.

INCOME

Many LGBTQ+ older adults end up working well past retirement age to support their cost of living. Approximately one-quarter to one-third of LGBTQ+ adults greater than 65 years old are living at or below 200% of the US federal poverty level with bisexual and transgender older adults even more adversely affected.[4,10] Studies also show that lesbian and bisexual older women are less likely to have health insurance than their heterosexual counterparts, further limiting access to health care.[10]

HEALTH CARE ELIGIBILITY

US law has greatly influenced access to health care. Before 2015, a same-sex marriage was not legal in all states thus limiting access to Medicare and Medicaid for partnered unemployed LGBTQ+ adults. To qualify for Medicare part A, one must work 40 quarters or must be married to a spouse that has worked for this time. It was not until the

Supreme Court ruling in 2015 that legalized same-sex marriage nationwide, Obergefell v Hodges, that this access became possible.[11] For partnered LGBTQ+ older adults that are not legally married, a significant financial burden can occur when one partner needs long-term care and there is no legal recognition of this relationship. If each partner is living separately but interdependently, the financial burden on the caregiving partner may be less apparent and marriage may or may not be of financial benefit. Disability status may also be a barrier to care. For LGBTQ+ older adults who are disabled and dependent on social benefits, the decision to marry may impact their eligibility leading to loss of both benefits and access to health care.

COST OF LONG-TERM CARE

The cost of additional caregiving support is a burdensome expense for all older adults. Medicare does not pay for long-term care in the home or in a long-term care facility. However, in one study in 2010, 57% of LGBTQ+ people surveyed incorrectly anticipated that Medicare would pay for long-term care as opposed to 49% of the general population, though understanding of Medicaid benefits was about the same.[12]

In-home support and long-term care benefits may be provided through Medicaid if a person qualifies. The decision to marry may change a person's health care benefits and Medicaid eligibility if incomes are combined. Even if In-Home Support Services are an option through Medicaid, the couple may be wary of inviting a stranger into the home for fear of needing to conceal their sexual or gender identity. In some cases, an individual unmarried partner may be forced to sell their home to pay for care in lieu of the protections of Medicaid for spousal impoverishment that permits the spouse to keep a percentage of the couple's income to continue living in the home. Without the protection of marriage, a partner would not be able to apply for Family Medical Leave Act to care for their loved one in a time of need. Even for married couples who qualify, the desire to protect privacy and to prevent accidental "outing" may lead to resistance to filing claims for social supports and anxiety regarding completing forms requesting information on next of kin.[8]

RETIREMENT

Older LGBTQ+ adults often end up working past retirement age without having the savings to retire comfortably or the means to pay for unanticipated expenses like the cost of care. The Aegon Center for Longevity and Retirement conducted an international survey of 900 LGBTQ+ workers and retired adults in Australia, Brazil, Canada, France, Germany, the Netherlands, Spain, and the United States.[9] Their study found that the income of LGBTQ+ households is approximately 8% lower than heterosexual counterparts with LGBTQ+ women having an income 17% less than their peers and 27% less than heterosexual men; 55% retired earlier than planned compared with 45% of heterosexual adults with poor health being a more common reason. According to the Met Life "Still Out Still Aging" study in 2010, 59% of the surveyed LGBT population reported having less than $50,000 in assets compared with 48% of the general respondents.[12]

SOCIAL SECURITY SURVIVORSHIP BENEFITS

After the 2015 Supreme Court ruling on same-sex marriage, LGBTQ+ spouses technically became eligible to receive social security survivor benefits when their partner died. However, the law remained that only surviving spouses who were more than 60 years old and had been legally married for 9 months would be eligible, disqualifying many LGBTQ+ adults living in states that did not recognize same-sex marriage before the ruling.[13] In November 2021, the Social Security Administration changed eligibility criteria so that surviving partners of same-sex marriages would qualify if they would have been married at the time of the partner's death and if they would have been married for a longer period if state law had permitted it.[13] This change in the law expanded benefit eligibility to same-sex married couples by eliminating this inequity surrounding marriage laws.

HOUSING

Disparities in finances and health make the need for safe and affordable housing imperative. Up until 2020, there were no federal housing protections based on sexual and gender identity, though there were laws passed at state and local levels.[14] LGBTQ+ older adults have been subject to discrimination from real estate agents, home sellers, property owners/management companies, mortgage lenders, county permitting officials, and neighbors without federal legal recourse. Discrimination may be in the form of blatant refusal to engage or more subtle by not offering to show a one-bedroom apartment to a same-sex couple, charging additional fees and requiring additional background checks. According to the Equal Rights Center and SAGE (Services and Advocacy for LGBTQ + Elders), 48% of same-sex couples who applied for senior housing experienced some form of discrimination.[13]

The Federal Fair Housing Law enacted in 1968 prohibited discrimination based on sex. Only with extensive advocacy had this been used to protect LGBTQ+ older adults as sex was not considered synonymous with gender identity and sexual orientation. In 2020, the law was changed to include both gender identity and sexual orientation allowing for investigation and action against discriminatory practices.

These challenges with housing have led to fewer LGBTQ+ older adults becoming homeowners compared with non-LGBTQ+ counterparts.[5] Those identifying as African American/Black, Hispanic/Latino, transgender and nonbinary and single are even less likely to be homeowners.[5]

HOUSING SOLUTIONS

Work has been done to create affordable and inclusive LGBTQ+ affirming senior housing, but options remain extremely limited.[9] There is also a movement to work on allowing sexual and gender minorities to age in place as desired by most older adults. However, given the magnified disparities in financial security, social connections, and mistrust of the health care system and social supports, significant advocacy for culturally competent care, the development of a community, and policies for discrimination are necessary first steps.[8]

ADVANCE CARE PLANNING DOCUMENTATION

Amy brings Yvette back to the doctor for a 6-month check-in. Yvette has had a few close calls with forgetting to turn off the stove after scrambling an egg and burning a frozen meal in the microwave. She has also become increasingly paranoid about her relationship with Amy and not wanting anyone to know her gender identity history or sexual orientation. She does not let the doctor undress her for the physical examination. The doctor asks the names of family members to update her "next of kin" given that Yvette is not married and asks Yvette for permission to contact her family. Yvette stays silent and gives Amy a panicked look. Amy spots a copy of an advance directive on the shelf on the room and picks a copy on the way out.

Advance directives are a set of legal documents that allows a person's wishes for their health and bodies to be specified in case they are unable to speak for themselves or lack decision-making capacity. According to multiple studies, LGBTQ+ older adults are generally more proactive at completing these documents compared with the general population especially when it comes to health care power of attorney documentation and hospital visitation documentation.[12,15]

HEALTH CARE POWER OF ATTORNEY/HEALTH CARE PROXY

These directives allow individuals to identify a health care power of attorney that would be able to uphold their wishes should they not be able to advocate for themselves.[16] Legally, states will designate an automatic "next of kin" to be the decision maker if no advance directive is available. "Next of kin" is traditionally a person's legal spouse, children, or parents. For many LGBTQ+ older adults that are no longer in contact or on good terms with their biological family or who do not have a legally recognized spouse, health care decisions could end up being made without taking their dignity or wishes into consideration. Completion of this advance directive allows LGBTQ+ adults to designate chosen family members as health care decision makers over legally recognized next of kin to uphold preferences stated in a living will.

LIVING WILL

The directive also includes a living will which states preferences for life-sustaining treatments. However, research into end-of-life decisions in LGBTQ+ adults show that the vast majority have not spoken to their primary care providers specifically about their preferences for end-of-life care as these conversations are not readily initiated by the health care system.[15]

ESTATE AND ASSET DISTRIBUTION PLANNING

A living trust or will are examples of estate planning documents that determine the distribution of assets and legal custody of children. If a person dies without a living trust, assets are distributed based on the state law of succession. For unmarried LGBTQ+ older adults who are financially interdependent, not completing this document could leave the surviving partner without financial assets.[17]

For people with life insurance or retirement plans, beneficiary designations can be specified to whom would receive the benefits. If property is owned, documents can be prepared with the help of a lawyer to ensure appropriate transfer of real estate ownership at the time of death.

UPHOLDING CORRECT NAMES AND PRONOUNS

For transgender older adults, "deadnaming" or calling a nonbinary person by a name they no longer use is an infraction on dignity. LGBTQ+ specific advance care planning documentation for transgender adults should include a directive upholding their correct name, pronouns, and gender identity at the end of life or if these individuals cannot speak for themselves.[18]

FUNERAL DIRECTIVE

Given that the power of attorney for health care terminates after a person dies, it is recommended that older LGBTQ+ adults complete a funeral directive which authorizes a designated decision maker to uphold preferences regarding funeral arrangements/disposition of remains after the time of death.[16]

HOSPITAL VISITATION DIRECTIVE

A hospital visitation directive allows an individual to state who can or cannot visit during a hospitalization which avoids the heteronormative and cisgender assumption of the rights of next of kin and could allow for legal precedence to avoid discrimination by health care workers that may not acknowledge chosen family as such.[16]

ADVANCE CARE PLANNING COMPLETION RATE

Although advance care planning seems to be especially important in this population, data show that living will and health care proxy documentation rates are low though may be higher than the general population.[15] Transgender adults have the lowest rates of advance care planning documentation completion with rates 50% to 70% lower than their LGB counterparts.[15] Although documentation rates are higher, end-of-life conversations and preferences for life-sustaining treatment end up occurring *outside* of the clinical setting.[19] There is a recognized paucity of data regarding advance care planning completion rates and how systemic discrimination has led to a lack of completion among sexual and gender minorities.[19] Current data suggest that health care systems could improve advance care planning in this population by creating an inclusive environment that is free of judgment and that has opportunities for training and a zero-tolerance policy for discrimination[19] (**Table 1**).

LONG-TERM CARE

Yvette begins to struggle with managing her meals while Amy is at work. Amy has deactivated the stove and microwave. Yvette starts to lose weight. One day, Amy finds her on the floor when she returns from work—it is unknown how long she had been down but she had soiled herself. Amy realizes that she cannot function alone anymore but is too afraid to ask for help. What if the home care agency is uncomfortable with LGBTQ+ people? What if they assault Yvette while she is away at work? What if they try to contact Yvette's estranged family? Amy does a search—does an LGBTQ+ affirming memory care exist?

The move toward accepting help in the home and moving to long-term care is a big step for any older adult and caregiver in terms of cost, concern for safety and finding the right community. For LGBTQ+ older adults, financial insecurity, isolation, and fear of discrimination lead to challenges in securing the right level of care. A study of LGBTQ+ older adults by Johnson and colleagues in 2005 found that 73% of respondents believed that discrimination exists in long-term care, 74% believed they do not include sexual discrimination in policies, 60% did not believe that they had equal access to social/health services, 34% believed they would have to hide their sexual orientation, and 98% stated that they would want a gay or gay-friendly housing option.[8]

LONG-TERM CARE EQUALITY INDEX

Recently, SAGE and the Human Rights Campaign Foundation developed the Long-Term Care Equality Index (LEI) to set national standards for inclusive policies and best practices along with a consumer's guide on how to evaluate long-term care options for sexual and gender minority-affirming living.[20] The guide provides step-by-step guidance for older adults and their caregivers on how to assess an agency

Table 1
Summary of advance care planning documents for LGBTQ+ older adults

Name	Definition	Importance for LGBTQ+ Older Adults
Advance Directive	A set of legal documents that allows a person's wishes for their health and bodies to be specified in case they are unable to speak for themselves or lack decision-making capacity	Completion helps LGBTQ+ adults maintain their dignity, uphold preferences, and ensure families of choice are protected financially at the end of life and postmortem
Healthcare Power of Attorney/Health Care Proxy	Designates a legal power of attorney to uphold wishes and/or make decisions related to health care	Legally permits family of choice over legally recognized next of kin to uphold and make health care-related decisions
Living Will	A document that states preferences for life-sustaining treatments	Assures that a person's individual wishes are upheld instead of relying on legal precedence that is biased by cultural norms
Living Trust/Will	An estate planning document that determines distribution of assets and legal custody of children	Supersedes legal precedence that would not recognize families of choice over next of kin
Directive to Uphold Name/Pronouns	A document that indicates a person's name and pronouns	LGBTQ+ older adults may not use the name given by their family of origin. This directive ensures that a person's chosen name and pronouns will be used if they are unable to speak for themselves
Funeral Directive	A document that authorizes a designated decision maker to uphold preferences regarding funeral arrangements and disposition of remains after death	Health care power of attorney expires after a person dies. This directive permits family of choice to uphold wishes postmortem
Hospital Visitation Directive	A document that allows an individual to state who can or cannot visit during a hospitalization	Avoids heteronormative and cisgender assumptions of the rights of next of kin that would keep families of choice from visiting or that would permit an unwanted visitor

or living community based on nondiscrimination policies and the wording of these policies, practices for community outreach, signs of inclusivity, visitor/rooming policies, and collection of sexual orientation and gender identity information. As of 2023, there were 200 long-term care sites participating in the LEI survey across 34 states allowing long-term care facilities of all types to access free education on culturally competent sexual and gender minority informed care.

Ideally, Amy uses the LEI to find an LGBTQ+ affirming assisted living community for Yvette that is on the way to work at the bakery and not too costly. Amy visits her every day. They consult with a lawyer to ensure all of their advance care planning documentation is in place. While life has changed, Amy is relieved to know that Yvette is safe and well cared for in a community that accepts every aspect of their identities. Amy is now able to care for her own physical and mental health while focusing on quality time with Yvette.

SUMMARY

The financial and psychosocial challenges of LGBTQ+ older adults arise out of a lifetime of marginalization and laws that are constantly in flux and not supportive of the needs of LGBTQ+ older adults. Although some disparities that this population faces are universal, many are further compounded by gender and sexual minority identities (bisexual, lesbian, gay, transgender) in addition to race, health, disability, and financial status. Social isolation comes in many forms ranging from the effects of systemic discrimination to a reinforced protective mechanism for survival. The lack of financial security stems from lower income levels, limitations on access to health care and affordable housing, and decreased accumulated wealth prompting LGBTQ+ people to work past the average retirement age while managing multiple responsibilities including the often overlooked role of caregiving. Advance care planning becomes essential for LGBTQ+ older adults to not only maintain their dignity and uphold preferences at the end of life but also ensure their families of choice are protected financially. When living independently is no longer an option, it is important to have resources for long-term care options that are safe and inclusive for this especially vulnerable population. Further research and education on the extent of disparity and demonstration of inclusive practices among clinicians, social workers, social support systems, and long-term care facilities are pathways to remedy the social and financial well-being of LGBTQIA+ older adults.

CLINICS CARE POINTS

- LGBTQ+ older adults are twice as likely to be single and live alone and four times less likely to have children than their heterosexual counterparts.
- Research indicates that over half of surveyed LGBTQ+ older adults feel socially isolated.
- Eighty-two percent of older adults in this community have experienced at least one episode of victimization including verbal threats, harassment, and physical assault with two-thirds experiencing at least three episodes in their lifetime.
- Many LGBTQ+ adults are thrown into the role of caregiving with 21% of older LGBTQ+ people providing care to a friend compared with just 6% of non-LGBTQ+ counterparts and without the same clinical, social, and financial resources to do so.
- One-quarter to one-third of LGBTQ+ adults greater than 65 years old are living at or below 200% of the US federal poverty level with bisexual and transgender older adults even more adversely affected.

- **LGBTQ+ older adults' household income is less than their gender and sexual majority counterparts, and they have less accumulated savings for retirement.**
- **Forty-eight percent of same-sex couples who applied for senior housing experienced some form of discrimination, which contributes to housing insecurity.**

ACKNOWLEDGMENTS

Marika Blair Humber, PhD; Chalise Carlson, MA.

DISCLOSURE

Views expressed in this article are those of the authors and not necessarily those of the Department of Veterans Affairs, the Federal Government, or TPMG. This work would not be possible without multiple collaborators, clinicians, and key partners.

REFERENCES

1. Goldsen KF. Shifting social context in the lives of LGBTQ older adults. Public Policy Aging Rep 2018;28(1):24–8.
2. Cacioppo S, Grippo AJ, London S, et al. Loneliness: clinical import and interventions. Perspect Psychol Sci 2015;10(2):238–49.
3. National Institute on Aging. What Do We Know About Healthy Aging? Published February 23, 2022. Accessed May 29, 2023. https://www.nia.nih.gov/health/what-do-we-know-about-healthy-aging#loneliness.
4. Sage, National Resource Center on LBGT Aging. Facts On LGBTQ+ Aging. Published online March 2021. https://www.sageusa.org/resource-posts/facts-on-lgbt-aging/.
5. Cantave C. Dignity 2022: the experience of LGBTQ older adults. AARP Research; 2022. https://doi.org/10.26419/res.00549.001.
6. LGBT Caregiver Concerns. Alzheimer's Association; 2014. Accessed June 26, 2023. https://www.lgbtagingcenter.org/resources/pdfs/caregiversAAbrochure.pdf.
7. Stinchcombe A, Smallbone J, Wilson K, et al. Healthcare and end-of-life needs of lesbian, gay, bisexual, and transgender (LGBT) older adults: a scoping review. Geriatrics 2017;2(1):13.
8. Addis S, Davies M, Greene G, et al. The health, social care and housing needs of lesbian, gay, bisexual and transgender older people: a review of the literature. Health Soc Care Community 2009;17(6):647–58.
9. Larkin M. Enhancing health, wellness and community. International Council on Active Aging®; 2018. https://www.icaa.cc/store_detail.php?id=6549. Accessed July 26, 2023.
10. Emlet CA. Social, economic, and health disparities among LGBT older adults. Generations. Journal of the American Society on Aging 2016;40(2):16–22. https://www.jstor.org/stable/26556193. Accessed May 22, 2023.
11. Sage. Marriage, Medicare & Medicaid: What Same-Sex Couples Need to Know. Published online 2023.https://www.lgbtagingcenter.org/resources/pdfs/SAGE%20SHIP%20Marriage%20Medicare%20Medicaid%20Final%20R1.pdf.
12. American Society on Aging, MetLife Mature Market Institute. Still Out Still Aging: The MetLife Study of Lesbian, Gay, Bisexual, and Transgender Baby Boomers. Published online 2010. https://www.asaging.org/sites/default/files/files/mmi-still-out-still-aging.pdf.

13. Salmon J. Social security expands survivor benefit eligibility for same-sex partners. AARP. 2022. Available at: https://www.aarp.org/retirement/social-security/info-2022/survivors-benefits-lgbtq-expansion.html. Accessed September 21, 2023.
14. Increasing LGBT Cultural Competence. sageusa.org/lgbthousing. https://www.sageusa.org/wp-content/uploads/2019/02/increasing-lgbt-cultural-competence-housing.pdf. Accessed May 22, 2023.
15. Kcomt L, Gorey KM. End-of-Life preparations among lesbian, gay, bisexual, and transgender people: integrative review of prevalent behaviors. J Soc Work End-of-Life Palliat Care 2017;13(4):284–301.
16. Sage. The Legal Documents Every LGBT Older Adult Needs. LGBTAgingCenter.org. Published April 2011. https://www.lgbtagingcenter.org/resources/resource.cfm?r=3. Accessed May 24, 2023.
17. Lin J. Estate planning considerations for LGBTQ couples. NOLO; 2023. https://www.nolo.com/legal-encyclopedia/six-key-estate-planning-issues-gay-lesbian-couples.html. Accessed June 26, 2023.
18. Prachnaik C. Creating End-of-Life Documents for Trans Individuals: An Advocate's Guide. Published online October 2014. https://www.lgbtagingcenter.org/resources/resource.cfm?r=694. Accessed July 26, 2023.
19. Reich AJ, Perez S, Fleming J, et al. Advance care planning experiences among sexual and gender minority people. JAMA Netw Open 2022;5(7):e2222993.
20. Human Rights Campaign Foundation, Sage. Long-Term Care Equality Index 2023. Published online 2023. https://www.lgbtagingcenter.org/resources/resource.cfm?r=1013.

Postacute Care and Long-term Care for LGBTQ+ Older Adults

Jennifer L. Carnahan, MD, MPH, MA[a,b,c,*],
Andrew C. Pickett, MSEd, PhD[d]

KEYWORDS

• Nursing home • Long-term care • Postacute care • LGBTQ+

KEY POINTS

- Social isolation, limited community supports, dementia, decreased functional abilities, economic limitations, and delays in care may all be reasons why an lesbian, gay, bisexual, transgender, queer + (LGBTQ+) older adult may be admitted to a nursing home.
- Cultivating an inclusive and LGBTQ + culturally competent nursing home culture means that all staff and clinicians should receive training specific to working with this group and time should be allocated for this to reduce staff burden.
- Although older adults fear being forced into the closet while in a nursing home, they also simultaneously fear unwanted disclosure of their sexual orientation or gender identity status, and their autonomy should be respected either way.

INTRODUCTION

More than 15,000 nursing homes in the United States provide rehabilitative and skilled nursing care to primarily older adults. Nursing homes originally served as homes for aging, often impoverished individuals who could no longer care for themselves at home.[1] This population could include unwed or childless women and individuals estranged from their family members.

Over time, nursing homes have become increasingly medicalized. The population of nursing home residents can be divided into 2 distinct groups: postacute care residents and long-term care residents. Of those insured by Medicare, postacute care residents

[a] Indiana University Center for Aging Research, Regenstrief Institute, 1101 West 10th Street, Indianapolis, IN 46202, USA; [b] Department of Medicine, Indiana University School of Medicine, Indianapolis, IN, USA; [c] Roudebush VA Medical Center, Indianapolis, IN, USA; [d] Department of Health & Wellness Design, Indiana University Bloomington, 1719 East 10th Street, Bloomington, IN 47408, USA
* Corresponding author. Department of Medicine, Indiana University School of Medicine, 1101 West 10th Street, Indianapolis, IN 46202.
E-mail address: jenncarn@iu.edu

Clin Geriatr Med 40 (2024) 321–331
https://doi.org/10.1016/j.cger.2023.10.005
0749-0690/24/Published by Elsevier Inc.

receiving temporary rehabilitative services bring in more funds to nursing homes via Medicare Part A payments.[2] They typically have greater acute medical and rehabilitative needs than long-term residents, requiring more highly skilled services, and are also susceptible to poor outcomes such as high mortality and readmissions rates.[3,4]

Some postacute care residents will convert to become long-term residents of nursing homes if they can no longer safely care for themselves at home or reside in the community. In addition to decreased functional ability, long-term nursing home residents usually have multiple chronic conditions. Most long-term care residents' nursing home care is eventually funded by state-run Medicaid plans once they are unable to pay out of pocket or via long-term care insurance for their care.[5] In 2022, on average, the primary payer source for 62% of nursing home residents in the United States was Medicaid, followed by private pay insurance or other sources (25%), with Medicare funding the remaining proportion of nursing home residents (13%).[6]

By virtue of requiring care in nursing homes, both postacute care residents and long-term residents rely on the support of nursing home staff and professionals for their day-to-day functions and medical care. This support need also increases nursing home residents and residents' vulnerability to negative outcomes when there are system failures or staffing issues compromising their care. This was evident during the early coronavirus disease 2019 pandemic when nursing home populations were decimated by the outbreak.[7] This support need also increases the vulnerability of marginalized populations in nursing homes, such as members of the LGBTQ + community. The following will examine the predisposing circumstances that lead LGBTQ + individuals to nursing homes, examine some of the experiences and needs of this population in nursing homes, and outline best practices and resources for culturally competent and inclusive care of LGBTQ + individuals in nursing homes.

LGBTQ + HEALTH CARE

Each letter in the acronym LGBTQ + stands for a subset of the population. Although older adults who identify as LGBTQ+ and receive care in nursing homes will be discussed in general, it is important to recognize that each subset may have their own specific supports and needs that should be considered individually.[8] The intersection of different potentially marginalizing characteristics or identities—age, reliance on others for daily functions, LGBTQ+, gender, economic disadvantage, race, and ethnicity—underscore the importance of respecting and acknowledging the individual person who is the resident in the nursing home.

Having lived through times when sexual orientation or gender identity (SOGI) minorities were criminalized and being closeted was often safer, LGBTQ + older adults may not self-identify to medical staff in nursing homes and other settings.[9] There are limited studies of LGBTQ + individuals living in nursing homes. Even in larger databases, there has historically been a "don't ask" approach to asking older adults demographic SOGI questions. For example, the Health and Retirement Study, a 30+-year longitudinal study of a cohort of more than 20,000 people in the United States aged 50 years and above, only began asking sexual orientation questions in 2016 and still does not identify whether participants are transgender.[10,11]

Because of this dearth of scholarship, some of the studies cited here draw on international work examining care for LGBTQ + older adults in nursing homes or nursing home approximations in international contexts. Other studies ask LGBTQ + elders how they perceive long-term care although they themselves are not necessarily long-term care residents yet. Finally, some studies examine care in assisted living or nursing homes without separating the two. That said, the nursing home perspective is prioritized in this article.

PREDISPOSING CIRCUMSTANCES FOR NURSING HOME ADMISSIONS

Several factors contribute to the decision for an older adult to enter care in a nursing home, regardless of SOGI status (**Fig. 1**). Limited ability to care for oneself and a lack of available care partners who can manage one's care needs combined with complex medical comorbidities, whether due to an acute illness or due to progression of a chronic illness, can lead to a nursing home admission.[12] Decreased ability to perform daily functions is also a cause of nursing home admission, short or long stay.[13] Many LGBTQ + people anticipate needing to rely on professional assistance for these self-care gaps.[14] Among the LGBTQ + population, there is evidence that there is a greater propensity to have reduced ability to perform activities of daily living (ADLs) and instrumental ADLs.[10,15] There is some evidence that stigma and ongoing microaggressions have a greater association with physical impairment in older generations of sexual and gender minorities (SGM).[16]

Social isolation and a limited care support network may also contribute to long-term care admission. Social isolation is a concerning trend among older adults and is magnified among the older LGBTQ + population.[17] This may be especially true for older LGBTQ + veterans.[18] Many members of the older LGBTQ + community have experienced estrangement from their families of origin. Coming out later in life may lead to estrangement from adult children who are therefore unavailable as caregivers.[19] A "chosen family" may serve a care partner role but may not consistently be legally recognized.[20,21] Similar to a family of origin, a chosen family may also eventually be limited in their ability to support the older adult aging in place.

Despite increased care needs, there is also a perception of limited access to supportive care services among SGM older adults.[22] Additionally, at least a third of LGBTQ + older adults report an income that is less than 200% below the US federal poverty level.[23] They may not be able to afford additional support at home and be more likely to turn to Medicaid-supported long-term care services, once they are

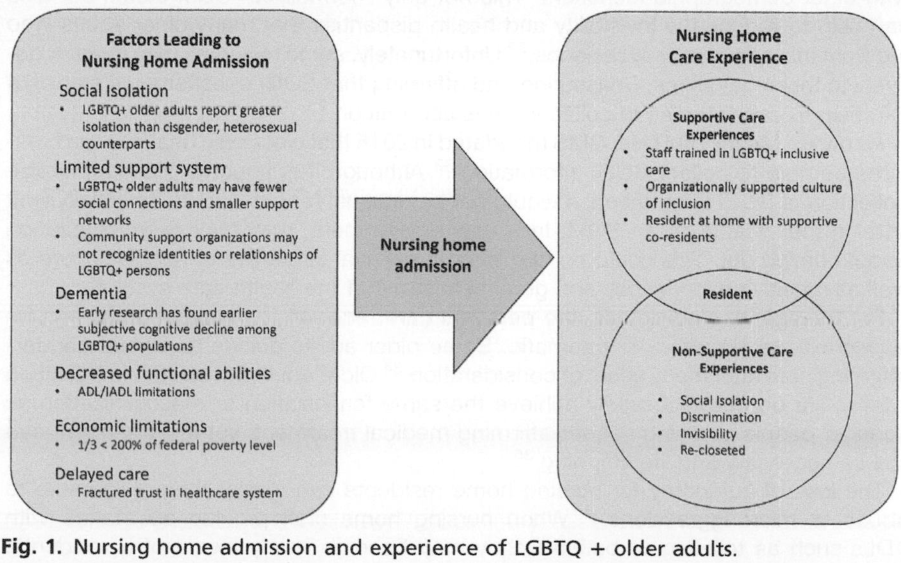

Fig. 1. Nursing home admission and experience of LGBTQ + older adults.

able to access them. Among some LGBTQ + older adults, there is a perception that long-term services and supports are unaffordable and thus unattainable, which may limit pursuit of these resources.[24] This naturally leads to requests for these services and supports when the need has been prolonged, a wait, which may contribute to an increased propensity for progression to nursing home admission.

Within nursing homes, approximately 50% of residents are living with dementia or some other type of cognitive impairment. Dementia can pose a particular fear for SGM older adults. Having faced discrimination, dementia poses the real possibility of being stripped of the identity that one fought so hard to accept.[24] Relatedly, individuals may forget to whom they have or have not disclosed SOGI details, and reasons for doing so. For example, among transgender residents with unsupportive families of origin who are the primary decision-makers, staff may be told to dress the resident in clothing that is incongruent with the resident's identity.[21] A dementia diagnosis increases the risk of elder abuse regardless of SOGI status.[25]

LGBTQ + individuals have higher incidence of cardiovascular risk factors that increase their risk of dementia; they also perceive themselves at a higher risk of dementia diagnosis than their cis-heterosexual counterparts.[26,27] Those who have endured greater discrimination may be at higher risk of dementia than those who have less traumatic life experiences.[28] The true risk of all-cause dementia may not be higher risk in the LGBTQ + population although limited data collection on SOGI status impairs researchers' ability to confirm this.[29,30] Regardless, SGM older adults at a minimum have the same risk of dementia as the general US population, and dementia increases the risk of nursing home admission.[31]

Dementia, delayed care, limited economic resources, limited support systems, decreased functional abilities, and social isolation all indicate that LGBTQ + elders are highly likely to require nursing home care.

NURSING HOME EXPERIENCES

When new residents are being admitted, whether they are either long term or short term, standard practice should be to ask SOGI questions of every new resident along with other demographic identifiers. This not only "normalizes" SGM status but also can help to reduce the invisibility and health disparities that many older adults who are from this community experience.[32] Unfortunately, some residents may react negatively to these questions. Reassuring and affirming that SOGI questions are standard can help to ease hurdles to collecting this information.[21]

As part of Meaningful Use, CMS mandated in 2015 that electronic health record systems be able to collect SOGI information.[33] Although it is important to standardize collection of SOGI information, it would not be unusual for older adults to initially limit sharing their status as an SGM. In a new environment, they may exercise caution about coming out. This could be due to both survival strategies of nondisclosure as well as negative experiences and general mistrust of the health-care system.

For transgender individuals, the personal care received in nursing homes can be supportive, as intended, or traumatic. Some older adults decide to pursue gender-affirming care after many years of consideration.[34] Older adults who begin to transition later in life do not necessarily achieve the same feminization or masculinization as younger people pursuing gender-affirming medical treatment, yet this treatment can still be necessary and life affirming.[35]

The loss of autonomy for nursing home residents can render them vulnerable to abuse or microaggressions.[13] When nursing home staff provide assistance with ADLs such as toileting or bathing, they may become newly aware of a resident's transgender status. If staff are not prepared for such an unintentional outing and how to react in a supportive manner they may demonstrate microaggressions. This biased reaction can be psychologically harmful for a transgender resident.[36]

Gay men who lived through the human immunodeficiency virus (HIV) epidemic can also mistrust health care after a lifetime of accumulated disappointments from homosexuality listed as a psychiatric disorder into the 1970s to the loss of friends and loved ones who died of acquired immunodeficiency syndrome (AIDS)-related complications during the 1980s and 1990s while experiencing inconsistent empathy from health-care providers.[37] Furthermore, transgender people often report a lack of access to adequate health-care providers.[38] These life course experiences will vary depending on which generation a resident falls within and with the intersection of a resident's various identities (eg, racial, gender, ethnic, family, education, or profession).

One survey found that only 22% of SGM older adults thought they could be out with long-term care providers.[39] Residents from different generations may have different degrees of comfort when it comes to disclosing their SGM status. Bisexual or questioning older adults may be less likely to disclose their SGM status and persons with higher income may be more likely to disclose their SGM status.[40] However, older adults are increasingly willing to disclose SOGI identities as societal acceptance increases.[9] One recent review found that various forms of social support were instrumental in disclosure of SOGI identity among older adults.[41] However, those in nursing home care may have limited access to their social networks, which may affect comfort with disclosure to staff and other residents.

Ultimately, if a resident feels unsafe due to their SGM status, this may exacerbate social isolation. Greater risk of mental health disorders goes hand in hand with SGM residents' risk of social isolation.[24] Residents may be reluctant to display photographs of their chosen family and loved ones or may even ask visitors to keep away to avoid being inadvertently outed.[24,42] Although degree of outness is the resident's decision, because outness has been linked to lower cortisol levels and better overall health, it is important to create a nursing home culture that helps the resident to feel safe and supported should they decide to come out.[43]

When cultivating a welcoming and inclusive culture in a nursing home, it is important to be aware that there will be different levels of comfort between residents. In particular, the word "queer" may be not appreciated or embraced by all SGM residents. Originally, a slur, queer, may have associations with unpleasant memories such as bullying or taunting for some residents. Non-SGM residents may continue to interpret queer as a slur and engage in bullying in nursing homes where inclusivity is not the cultural norm.[44]

Older adults who have been bullied or brutalized because of their SGM identify are at risk of posttraumatic stress disorder if they are not well supported in their long-term care community. Women, in particular, may have safety concerns from living in a nursing home and the autonomy that is relinquished there.[45] Many nursing homes are affiliated with religious organizations, which can also be triggering for some LGBTQ + people. Furthermore, current news and national climate toward LGBTQ + people may exacerbate or trigger a trauma response. After decades of consistent growth in acceptance, recent national polling has seen plateaus, and even minor declines, in the overall acceptance of SGM persons and relationships.[46] Televisions are ubiquitous in many nursing homes, with news of current events broadcast. Residents with visual or ambulatory impairments may have difficulty changing the channel or volume level. A trauma-informed care approach can ameliorate and protect against traumatic triggers for SGM residents.[42,47]

A 2018 survey by the AARP (formerly American Association of Retired Persons) found that when considering admission to a nursing home, most SGM older adults anticipate neglect, abuse, refusal of services, harassment, and being forced back into the closet.[48] Fear of abuse and stigmatization may be related to the resident's own personal story. Some staff may be resistant to additional training in SGM inclusivity arguing that they treat "everyone the same."[49] This approach can be harmful and invalidating by not acknowledging a vital component of a resident's identity. An important distinction in considering older adults' trepidation regarding nursing homes is identifying the difference between fear of being forced into the closet and invisibility.[45,50] Being forced into the closet is a survival technique for safety, whereas invisibility occurs when a predominant cis-heterosexual culture assumes LGBTQ + residents do not exist. Neither is ideal but by treating all residents the same, rather than reducing health disparities, this approach may instead ignore the unique life stories and identities of residents from further marginalizing them.

Some of the same factors that contributed to a nursing home admission can also create barriers to suitable care in the nursing home. Health-care workers across disciplines are not well trained in care for LGBTQ + older adults. Stereotypes and inadequate knowledge of the LGBTQ + population are not uncommon among those who care for older adults.[22,51] For example, when confronted with consensual sexual

Table 1
Best practice recommendations for nursing home

Practice Area	Recommendations
SOGI identifiers	*Ask SOGI questions at admission along with other demographic identifiers
Medications	*Consider medications, especially gender affirming medications, in light of the resident's specific goals and priorities *Ensure labs for any HIV medications can be collected and analyzed in a timely manner
Social isolation	*Do not force residents to be out but support them in having chosen family visit, displaying photographs, and expressing their authentic selves
Inclusive culture	*Set institutional standards of inclusivity *Display inclusive imagery or displays prominently
Staff training	*All staff should have protected time set aside for training including administrative and frontline *Engage with one of the resources listed in **Table 2** for training
Trauma-informed care	*Trauma-informed care is mandated in US Nursing Homes *Train staff to recognize residents with trauma history *Support residents with trauma history through staff trainings on trauma-informed care
Advance care planning and surrogate decision making	*Update the Health care Power of Attorney *When identifying surrogate decision-makers use nonspecific language such as "who do you rely on for help at home?" rather than assuming family of origin will be involved *Use the Rainbow PELI tool to identify care preferences (see **Table 2**) *For long stay residents fill out a POLST form

Abbreviations: POLST, physician orders for life sustaining treatment.

Table 2
Resource list

Resource	Description
https://www.hrc.org/resources/long-term-care facilities	The Long-term Care Equality Index is a tool that the Human Rights Campaign and SAGE compiled that enables the user to search for LGBTQ + friendly senior communities, assisted living, and nursing homes. They provide information on how to qualify for listing in the index
https://www.preferencebasedliving.com/	The Rainbow PELI and other tools from Preference Based Living are designed specifically to help long-term care staff identify an LGBTQ + resident's care preferences. Some questions align with MDS mandated assessments
https://www.sageusa.org/	SAGE is an organization located in New York City that supports and advocates for LGBTQ + older adults across the United States. They collaborate with other organizations to provide services to this population. Educational materials can be found here
https://www.lgbtagingcenter.org/	The National Resource Center on LGBTQ + Aging provides educational materials and trainings on LGBTQ + older adults, state specific resources, and other technical assistance
https://www.outcarehealth.org/	Outcare Health provides educational opportunities and listings of LGBTQ + friendly providers
https://www.patientcare.va.gov/LGBT/index.asp	The VA provides resources for LGBTQ + veterans at every health center. Experts in trauma-informed care, the VA can provide additional supports to residents who are veterans
Welcoming LGBT Residents: A Practical Guide for Senior Living Staff	This book by Tim R. Johnston provides invaluable insights into every aspect of promoting an inclusive and culturally competent care for LGBTQ + nursing home residents. It contains practical advice as well as detailed information on how to best care for this population

Abbreviations: MDS, minimum data set; VA, United States Department of Veterans Affairs.

relations between 2 LGBTQ + residents, staff may assume the behavior is inherently deviant.[52] Nursing home policies regarding sexual activity of residents should be applied equitably with understanding that same sex relations may occur, even among residents assumed to be heterosexual.[36] Training programs that engage nursing home staff in LGBTQ + cultural competency can remediate staff knowledge and ensure more equitable care.

Just as an LGBTQ + resident faces potential stigmatization from nursing home staff, they also face stigmatization from other residents. At the same time, it is paramount that staff and nursing home administrators not assume that most residents will be prejudiced against SGM residents.[44] Although non-SGM older adults have the potential for homophobia and transphobia, assuming an older generation will resist LGBTQ + inclusivity reflects an implicit ageism.

Finally, it is essential that legal planning and advance care planning are implemented with SGM older adults. Lack of awareness of the priorities of persons living in long-term care runs the risk of providing care that is not consistent with their goals and needs. Given their susceptibility to social isolation and potential desire to enlist chosen rather than biological family, nursing home social workers or case managers should prioritize clear establishment of residents' wishes. Otherwise, state laws will dictate who surrogate decision-makers are should the resident be unable to make their own medical decisions.[20] Using language that does not make assumptions about a family of origin can help to elicit essential information about who they prefer to make these decisions and how they would prefer them to be made.

BEST PRACTICES

In a study of more than 700 older LGBTQ + adults in the US South, 76.3% of respondents indicated they would be more likely to use long-term care if the care were provided by an LGBTQ + individual.[40] Other studies asking similar questions about willingness to use long-term care have found that preferences vary with some SGM older adults reluctantly assuming they will require some form of long-term-care 1 day and others preferring it.[12,53] Some SGM adults question whether they wish to segregate themselves in nursing homes or communities that cater to the LGBTQ + population or not. Regardless, there are very few nursing homes that are designed primarily to serve the LGBTQ + community, and for most, it is untenable to expect to receive care in such specialized nursing homes. We offer the following best practice recommendations for nursing homes to create inclusive and welcoming environments (**Table 1**) and resources to enable acting on the recommendations (**Table 2**).

CLINICS CARE POINTS

- Collection of SOGI information should be a standard part of the nursing home admission process.
- Advance care planning and assistance with legal recognition of a nursing home resident's preferred surrogate decision-makers can help to ensure equitable care for LGBTQ + older adults.
- When caring for older adults who identify as LGBTQ+, nursing home staff may need to use trauma-informed care best practices.

DISCLOSURE

Funding: Dr J. L. Carnahan was supported by the National Institute on Aging, United States division of the National Institutes of Health [Grant K23AG062797].

ACKNOWLEDGMENTS

The views expressed in this article are those of the authors and do not necessarily represent the views of the US Department of Veterans Affairs.

REFERENCES

1. Vladeck BC. Unloving care: the nursing home tragedy. Basic Books; 1980. p. 305.
2. David S, Sheikh F, Mahajan D, Greenough W, Bellantoni M. Whom Do We Serve? Describing the target population for post-acute and long-term care, focusing on nursing facility, settings, in the era of population health. AMDA: The Society for Post-Acute and Long-Term Care Medicine; 2016. http://www.paltc.org/amda-

white-papers-and-resolution-position-statements/whom-do-we-serve-describing-target-population.

3. Allen LA, Hernandez AF, Peterson ED, et al. Discharge to a skilled nursing facility and subsequent clinical outcomes among older patients hospitalized for heart failure. Research Support, Non-U.S. Gov't Research Support, U.S. Gov't, P.H.S. Circulation. Heart Fail 2011;4(3):293–300.
4. Toles M, Anderson RA, Massing M, et al. Restarting the cycle: incidence and predictors of first acute care use after nursing home discharge. J Am Geriatr Soc 2014;62(1):79–85.
5. Issue Brief: Estimates of Medicaid Nursing Facility Payments Relative to Costs (MACPAC) (2023).
6. KFF. Distribution of Certified Nursing Facility Residents by Primary Payer Source. Accessed August 18, 2023. Available at: https://www.kff.org/other/state-indicator/distribution-of-certified-nursing-facilities-by-primary-payer-source/?currentTimeframe=0&sortModel=%7B%22colId%22:%22Location%22,%22sort%22:%22asc%22%7D.
7. Carnahan JL, Lieb KM, Albert L, et al. COVID-19 disease trajectories among nursing home residents. J Am Geriatr Soc 2021;69(9):2412–8.
8. Lintott L, Beringer R, Do A, et al. A rapid review of end-of-life needs in the LGBTQ+ community and recommendations for clinicians. Palliat Med 2022;36(4):609–24.
9. Goldsen KF. Shifting social context in the lives of LGBTQ older adults. Public Policy & Aging Report 2018;28(1):24–8.
10. Travers JL, Shippee TP, Flatt JD, et al. Functional limitations and access to long-term services and supports among sexual minority older adults. J Appl Gerontol 2022;41(9):2056–62.
11. Hanes DW, Clouston SAP. Ask again: including gender identity in longitudinal studies of aging. Gerontol 2020. https://doi.org/10.1093/geront/gnaa107.
12. Buczak-Stec E, König HH, Feddern L, et al. Long-term care preferences and sexual orientation-A systematic review and meta-analysis. J Am Med Dir Assoc 2023;24(3):331–42.e1.
13. Carnahan JL, Inger L, Rawl SM, et al. Complex transitions from skilled nursing facility to home: patient and caregiver perspectives. J Gen Intern Med 2021;36(5):1189–96.
14. Henning-Smith C, Gonzales G, Shippee TP. Differences by sexual orientation in expectations about future long-term care needs among adults 40 to 65 Years old. Am J Publ Health 2015;105(11):2359–65.
15. Hiedemann B, Brodoff L. Increased risks of needing long-term care among older adults living with same-sex partners. Am J Publ Health 2013;103(8):e27–33.
16. Fredriksen Goldsen K, Kim HJ, Jung H, et al. The evolution of aging with pride-national health, aging, and sexuality/gender study: illuminating the iridescent life course of LGBTQ adults aged 80 Years and older in the United States. Int J Aging Hum Dev 2019;88(4):380–404.
17. Wilson K, Kortes-Miller K, Stinchcombe A. Staying out of the closet: LGBT older adults' hopes and fears in considering end-of-life. Canadian journal on aging = La revue canadienne du vieillissement 2018;37(1):22–31.
18. Monin JK, Mota N, Levy B, et al. Older age associated with mental health resiliency in sexual minority US Veterans. Am J Geriatr Psychiatr 2017;25(1):81–90.
19. Anderson JG, Flatt JD, Cicero EC, et al. Inclusive care practices and policies among sexual and gender minority older adults. J Gerontol Nurs 2022;48(12):6–15.

20. Torke AM, Carnahan JL. Optimizing the clinical care of lesbian, gay, bisexual, and transgender older adults. JAMA Intern Med 2017;177(12):1715–6.
21. Johnston TR. Welcoming LGBT residents : a practical guide for senior living staff.
22. Caceres BA, Travers J, Primiano JE, et al. Provider and LGBT individuals' perspectives on LGBT issues in long-term care: a systematic review. Gerontol 2020;60(3): e169–83.
23. Fredriksen-Goldsen KI, Kim H-J, Bryan AEB, et al. The cascading effects of marginalization and pathways of resilience in attaining good health among LGBT older adults. Gerontol 2017;57(suppl_1):S72–83.
24. Putney JM, Keary S, Hebert N, et al. "Fear runs deep:" the anticipated needs of LGBT older adults in long-term care. J Gerontol Soc Work 2018;61(8):887–907.
25. Rogers MM, Storey JE, Galloway S. Elder mistreatment and dementia: a comparison of people with and without dementia across the prevalence of abuse. J Appl Gerontol 2023;42(5):909–18.
26. Flatt JD, Johnson JK, Karpiak SE, et al. Correlates of subjective cognitive decline in lesbian, gay, bisexual, and transgender older adults. J Alzheim Dis 2018;64(1): 91–102.
27. Caceres BA, Brody A, Luscombe RE, et al. A systematic review of cardiovascular disease in sexual minorities. Am J Publ Health 2017;107(4):e13–21.
28. Lambrou NH, Gleason CE, Obedin-Maliver J, et al. Subjective cognitive decline associated with discrimination in medical settings among transgender and nonbinary older adults. Int J Environ Res Publ Health 2022;19(15). https://doi.org/10.3390/ijerph19159168.
29. Perales-Puchalt J, Gauthreaux K, Flatt J, et al. Risk of dementia and mild cognitive impairment among older adults in same-sex relationships. Int J Geriatr Psychiatr 2019;34(6):828–35.
30. May JT, Myers J, Noonan D, et al. A call to action to improve the completeness of older adult sexual and gender minority data in electronic health records. J Am Med Inf Assoc : JAMIA 2023. https://doi.org/10.1093/jamia/ocad130.
31. Gaugler JE, Duval S, Anderson KA, et al. Predicting nursing home admission in the U.S: a meta-analysis. BMC Geriatr 2007;7:13.
32. Bosse JD, Leblanc RG, Jackman K, et al. Benefits of implementing and improving collection of sexual orientation and gender identity data in electronic health records. Comput Inform Nurs 2018;36(6):267–74.
33. Cahill SR, Baker K, Deutsch MB, et al. Inclusion of sexual orientation and gender identity in stage 3 meaningful use guidelines: a huge step forward for LGBT health. LGBT Health 2016;3(2):100–2.
34. Fabbre VD. Agency and social forces in the life course: the case of gender transitions in later life. J Gerontol B Psychol Sci Soc Sci 2017;72(3):479–87.
35. Hughto JMW, Gunn HA, Rood BA, et al. Social and medical gender affirmation experiences are inversely associated with mental health problems in a U.S. Non-probability sample of transgender adults. Arch Sex Behav 2020;49(7):2635–47.
36. Villar F, Faba J. Older people living in long term care: no place for sex?. In: Simpson P, editor. Desexualisation in Later Life: the limits of sex and intimacy. Policy Press; 2021. p. 163–70, chap 9. Sex and Intimacy in Later Life.
37. Cochrane M. When AIDS began : San Francisco and the making of an epidemic. New York: Routledge; 2004.
38. Lee JL, Huffman M, Rattray NA, et al. "I don't want to spend the rest of my life only going to a gender wellness clinic": healthcare experiences of patients of a comprehensive transgender clinic. J Gen Intern Med 2022;1–8.

39. (NSCLC) NSCLC. LGBT older adults in long-term care facilities: Stories from the field. National Research Center on LGBT Aging; 2011. Available at: https://www.lgbtagingcenter.org/resources/pdfs/NSCLC_LGBT_report.pdf.
40. Dickson L, Bunting S, Nanna A, et al. Older lesbian, gay, bisexual, transgender, and queer adults' experiences with discrimination and impacts on expectations for long-term care: results of a survey in the southern United States. J Appl Gerontol 2022;41(3):650–60.
41. Loeb AJ, Wardell D, Johnson CM. Coping and healthcare utilization in LGBTQ older adults: a systematic review. Geriatr Nurs 2021;42(4):833–42. New York, NY.
42. Robertson ML, Carnahan JL, Streed CG Jr. Caring for LGBTQ+ older adults at home. J Gen Intern Med 2023;38(6):1538–40.
43. Juster RP, Smith NG, Ouellet É, et al. Sexual orientation and disclosure in relation to psychiatric symptoms, diurnal cortisol, and allostatic load. Psychosom Med 2013;75(2):103–16.
44. Sussman T, Brotman S, MacIntosh H, et al. Supporting lesbian, gay, bisexual, & transgender inclusivity in long-term care homes: a Canadian perspective. Canadian journal on aging = La revue canadienne du vieillissement 2018;37(2):121–32.
45. Westwood S. 'We see it as being heterosexualised, being put into a care home': gender, sexuality and housing/care preferences among older LGB individuals in the UK. Health Soc Care Community 2016;24(6):e155–63.
46. Organization G. LGBTQ+ Rights. https://news.gallup.com/poll/1651/gay-lesbian-rights.aspx
47. O'Malley KA, Sullivan JL, Mills W, et al. Trauma-informed care in long-term care settings: from policy to practice. Gerontol 2022;63(5):803–11.
48. Houghton A. *Maintaining Dignity: Understanding and Responding to the Challenges Facing Older LGBT Americans*. Washington, DC: AARP Research; 2018. https://doi.org/10.26419/res.00217.001.
49. Fasullo K, McIntosh E, Buchholz SW, et al. LGBTQ older adults in long-term care settings: an integrative review to inform best practices. Clin Gerontol 2022;45(5): 1087–102.
50. Willis P, Almack K, Hafford-Letchfield T, et al. Turning the Co-production corner: methodological reflections from an action research project to promote LGBT inclusion in care homes for older people. Int J Environ Res Publ Health 2018;15(4):695.
51. May JT, Rainbow JG. A qualitative description of direct care workers of lesbian, gay, bisexual, transgender older adults. J Appl Gerontol 2023;42(4):597–606.
52. Cook C, Schouten V, Henrickson M, et al. Ethics, intimacy and sexuality in aged care. J Adv Nurs 2017;73(12):3017–27.
53. Singleton M, Adams MA, Poteat T. Older black lesbians' needs and expectations in relation to long-term care facility use. Int J Environ Res Publ Health 2022;(22): 19. https://doi.org/10.3390/ijerph192215336.

End-Of-Life and Palliative Care for Lesbian, Gay, Bisexual, Transgender, Queer or Questioning, or Another Diverse Gender Identity Older Adults

Evie Kalmar, MD, MS[a], Jeffrey Mariano, MD[b,*]

KEYWORDS

• Palliative care • Hospice • End of life • LGBTQ

KEY POINTS

- Palliative care is a type of specialized medical care for people living with serious illness.
- A history of trauma or discrimination in life and in health care can lead to avoidance or reluctance to receive care at the end of life.
- Lesbian, gay, bisexual, transgender, queer or questioning, or another diverse gender identity (LGBTQ+) people are more likely to have alternative family structures. It is important to engage in advance care planning to understand their values, clarify surrogate decision makers, and contribute to goal-concordant care at the end of life.
- Clinicians can follow recommendations in this article to ensure they are providing LGBTQ-inclusive palliative and hospice care.

INTRODUCTION

What Is Palliative Care?

Palliative care is a type of specialized medical care for people living with serious illness. Historically, palliative care focused on people with cancer, but it increasingly is available for people with other serious diagnoses such as dementia, heart failure, and chronic obstructive pulmonary disease. The goal of palliative care is to improve quality of life by providing support and relief with both the symptoms related to serious

[a] University of California, San Francisco, San Francisco Veterans Affairs Health, 4150 Clement Street, 181-G, San Francisco, CA 94121, USA; [b] Department of Geriatrics and Palliative Medicine, AGSF, Southern California Permanente Medical Group, Bernard J Tyson Kaiser Permanente School of Medicine, Kaiser Permanente West Los Angeles, 6041 Cadillac Avenue Module 150, Los Angeles, CA 90034, USA
* Corresponding author.
E-mail address: Jeffrey.D.Mariano@kp.org

Clin Geriatr Med 40 (2024) 333–345
https://doi.org/10.1016/j.cger.2023.11.004
0749-0690/24/Published by Elsevier Inc.

illness as well as the stress often associated with it. It is sometimes described as an extra layer of support. Unlike hospice care, which is a benefit for people in their last 6 months of life, palliative care can be provided at any stage of illness, including right after diagnosis.

Palliative care is provided by multidisciplinary teams, often including doctors, nurses, social workers, chaplains, and pharmacists. It can be provided to people in their homes, in the hospital, and other settings of care (ie, assisted living facilities, board and care homes). Good palliative care focuses on getting to know patients as people and understanding their values and what makes life worth living. This focus helps provide holistic, comprehensive care that is tailored to the individual. Beyond clinical care, palliative medicine looks to better understand, connect, and support not only the patient but also their support network.

The philosophy of palliative care aligns with providing high-quality, patient-centered, and trauma-informed care to lesbian, gay, bisexual, transgender, queer or questioning, or another diverse gender identity (LGBTQ+) people. As Kimberly Acquaviva[1] wrote in her book *LGBTQ-Inclusive Hospice and Palliative Care*, the goal should be to "shift from providing *special* care to LGBTQ+ people to instead providing *inclusive* care to *all* people, including those who are LGBTQ+." This does not mean treating everyone the same but, instead, means creating space for, respecting, and incorporating differences into care plans using cultural humility.

Locations of palliative care

Palliative care can be provided anywhere, though there distinguishing factors between primary and specialty palliative care. Primary palliative care refers to when palliative care elements such as advance care planning, assessing and management symptoms are completed by the primary care team or specialists.[2] Specialty palliative care refers to when palliative care is delivered by dedicated teams trained in palliative care. Many hospitals have inpatient palliative care consult teams. Increasingly, outpatient clinics offer specialty palliative care in clinic, by phone, and by video, which helps to support people in earlier stages of serious illness. Hospice care, which focuses on comfort and quality of life for people with a prognosis of less than 6 months, can also be provided in many settings.

The vast majority of people receiving hospice care receive it in their home through a home-visiting interdisciplinary hospice team. There are also options for hospice care in skilled nursing facilities and in dedicated hospice facilities for people whose care or symptom needs are greater than can be managed at home. As people with serious illnesses experience disease progression, they may transition from outpatient palliative care and other alternative home-based palliative/home visit programs to hospice, whetherhome or inpatient. For older LGBTQ+ adults, these transitions often involve meeting and establishing trust with a new health care team and a reluctance to enter long-term care facilities or other settings fearing they would need to conceal their sexual and/or gender identities to prevent discrimination.

Background of lesbian, gay, bisexual, transgender, queer or questioning, or another diverse gender identity people and palliative care

People's experience with serious illness is deeply influenced by their prior experiences with health care. In the case of LGBTQ+ individuals, it is unfortunately common to have experienced discrimination or bias in health care that may make people reluctant to seek needed care. This makes it that much more important to provide LGBTQ+-inclusive palliative care to create an environment where everyone feels safe and able to access palliative care. Even as recently as 2023, there are studies demonstrating that LGBT patients receiving palliative care were faced with inadequate, disrespectful, and even abusive care, even higher amongst transgender and gender diverse people.[3,4]

Family of choice and advance care planning

LGBTQ+ people are more likely to create their own families, choosing their family members in families of choice. A family of choice is one that is inclusive and based on emotional relationships, rather than only on legally recognized or biological relationships. LGBTQ+ older adults are more likely to be unpartnered, not have biological children, and live alone compared to the general population.[5] It was not until 2015 after the Supreme Court overturned the Defense of Marriage Act that marriage was legal for same sex couples in all 50 states. Before this, there was not a legal pathway to be recognized as a family for many LGBTQ+ couples. Historically, this meant many could be denied benefits or even visits from the next of kin who were not legally recognized. The implications of this denial of equality and discrimination faced by older LGBTQ+ adults cannot be overstated, particularly because it influences their interactions with health care to this day.

The fact that LGBTQ+ people are more likely to have alternative family structures highlights the importance of advance care planning and especially designation of a surrogate decision maker. Advance care planning is the process by which an individual can: 1) designate who they would trust to make medical decisions on their behalf if they no longer were able to do so themselves and 2) indicate their values and preferences around health care. This process can be important for everyone with serious illness and especially people who want to designate a nonfamily member to be their decision maker. Though it differs from state to state, most default hierarchies for surrogate decision makers are based on next of kin, prioritizing biological or legal family. Unfortunately, the rate of advance care planning remains low in the LGBTQ+ population, with one study from 2006 demonstrating that fewer than half of the people surveyed had an advance directive or durable power of attorney for health care.[6]

Considerations

LGBTQ+ people face unique challenges while receiving palliative care and hospice services. Studies have shown LGBTQ+ cohort experience lower quality of care and there is a dearth of literature on experience of LGBTQ+ patients and their family members receiving hospice care.[7]

Barriers to care

Systemic barriers occur at the systems level (representing systems, institutions, and services) and the individual level (characteristics directly impacting those seeking care), and combined, they provide a barrier to LGBTQ+ wishing to access end-of-life care. Some examples of these barriers are described in **Table 1**.

Intersectionality

The heterogeneity of LGBTQ+ older adults across populations, countries, and cultures highlights the important role of intersectionality. Intersectionality can be defined as the interconnected nature of social categorizations applied to a given individual or group, that creates overlapping and interdependent systems of discrimination, disadvantage, and marginalization. This can be sociopolitical and personal and, unfortunately, may also lead to internalized negative feelings associated with identity, such as internalized homophobia.

Table 1
Potential barriers to palliative and hospice care

Potential Health Care Organization Barriers	Potential Consequences
Heterosexist assumptions of patient's sexual and gender identity	Lack of inclusion of families of choice in decision-making
Lack of provider training about caring for SGM patients	SGM patients' needs may not be understood, and they may experience bias from their provider (conscious or unconscious)
Lack of culturally competent caregiver support and bereavement groups	Higher levels of caregiver strain and disenfranchised grief
Lack of integration and availability of resources for SGM people	Lower levels of satisfaction with care
Potential sexual and gender minority barriers	Potential consequences
Estrangement from family of origin	Incorrect assumptions in regard to surrogate decision-making
Higher rates of mistrust of health care systems	Delayed uptake of medical care
Nondisclosure of SGM status	Higher levels of disease-associated distress
Fear of discrimination by health care providers	Nondisclosure of SGM status and need to distance from friends and community
Complexity of relationship with religious-based organizations	Delayed access to care; reluctance to use pastoral care resources
Isolation and lack of social support	Greater levels of disease-associated distress
Potential societal, health care insurance, and legal barriers	Potential consequences
Variability in and potential fragility of legal protections	Loss of access of SGM spouses or partners to health care insurance
Lack of comprehensive legal protections	Child custody not formalized; burial rights for transgender individuals not observed

Abbreviation: SGM, sexual and gender minority.

From Maingi S, Bagabag AE, O'Mahony S. Current Best Practices for Sexual and Gender Minorities in Hospice and Palliative Care Settings. J Pain Symptom Manage. 2018 May;55(5):1420-1427. https://doi.org/10.1016/j.jpainsymman.2017.12.479. Epub 2017 Dec 27. PMID: 29288882, with permission

By acknowledging intersectionality, we can understand its impact in the experience of receiving health care and palliative and end-of-life care.

One framework for evaluating intersectionality is the ADDRESSING mnemonic, demonstrated in **Box 1**.[8] Intersectionality and cultural humility are reinforced when clinicians are open to attending to the many complexities of intergroup and intragroup differences. Only the patient can tell you which sets of identities are most salient to them and in what ways (for more on cultural humility and affirming care, please see N.M. Javier & R. Noy's, "Affirming Care for LGBTQ+ Patients", in this issue).

To illustrate the point of intersectionality within the LGBTQ+ population, consider the identity "Gay Asian American." This term encompasses numerous religious, geographic, acculturation levels as reflected in the ADDRESSING mnemonic. Thus, there is no such thing as a homogeneous LGBTQ+ Asian American approach to end-of-life decision-making. Culture and intersectionality *inform* decision-making but does not *determine* it.

Serious and progressive illness create priorities at the end of life that may be universal.[9] These include comfort and not being in pain, good communication between

Box 1
ADDRESSING mnemonic for elements of culture and intersectionality

- Age and cohort effects
- Degree of physical ability
- Degree of cognitive ability
- Religion
- Ethnicity and race
- Socioeconomic status
- Sexual orientation and gender identity
- Individualistic life experiences (such as trauma or level of acculturation)
- National origin
- Gender role expectations

patient and clinicians, maintaining hope, honoring spiritual beliefs, fixing relationships, making plans, and saying goodbye. These human values, however, are also colored by a wide array of intercultural and intracultural variations. It is only by asking about culture, identity, and values that we can begin to understand a person and provide patient-centered care.

Case Presentation

Mr S is an 80-year-old male who was recently diagnosed with stage IV non-small cell lung cancer with metastases to brain. He is at his outpatient palliative care clinic appointment.

His chief complaints are worsening memory, pain, anorexia, and weight loss. He is accompanied by Mr P, a 66-year-old Filipinx male, who is his partner of 15 years. The palliative care nurse commented to Mr P, "You are doing such a great job taking care of him. Are you a nurse? Also your English is so good. Where are you from? Is there someone else who makes decisions for him if he were unable?" He did not correct her.

Minority Stress

The case presentation illustrates "minority stress," the excess stress that individuals from stigmatized social categories are exposed to because of their social minority position. One definition of minority stress widely used is "the chronic, cumulative stress associated with stigma, due to objective events such as discrimination and victimization and psychological responses to these events such as internalized shame."[10–12] The cumulative stress caused by stigma and social marginalization is a set up for chronic stress and related health problems.

Microaggressions

Microaggressions are brief verbal, behavioral, or environmental indignities, whether intentional or unintentional, that communicate hostile, derogatory, or negative slights and insults. They also can fracture patient-provider relationships and limit the trust that is so important in palliative care relationships.

It is important to recognize that by the time a person is engaging with palliative care, they likely have a long history of experiencing microaggressions and this can impact their openness to care.

Clinical Pearl

Microaggressions often occur toward people of sexual and gender minorities and can negatively impact people's openness to care, even at the end of life.

These include

- Endorsement of heteronormative or gender normative culture and behaviors (eg, assuming someone of the opposite sex is a patient's partner in a family meeting rather than asking for introductions and relationship to the patient)
- Discomfort or disapproval of LGBTQ+ experiences
- Assumption of a universal LGBTQ+ experience (eg, assuming an LGBTQ+ patient on hospice does not have any children or that sexual orientation is a big part of who they are)
- Exoticization
- Denial of the reality of heterosexism and genderism (eg, not asking about someone's experience of prejudice or trauma related to their identities)
- Assumption about someone's sexual orientation or gender identity based on appearances (eg, assuming someone who has a partner of the opposite gender is heterosexual when in fact they may be bisexual)

Case Continued

Mr S was hospitalized after a seizure and the inpatient palliative care team was consulted. The inpatient team recommended discharge to a skilled nursing facility for rehabilitation. Mr S discussed this with Mr P and their friends. They recognized that he was weaker and might need more care than at home, but he ultimately declined referral to the skilled nursing facility based on the negative experience of a friend who died in a nursing facility during the acquired immune deficiency syndrome (AIDS) epidemic.

Social Safety

Social safety refers to reliable social connection, inclusion, protection, and degree of social belonging, which are core human needs that are imperiled by societal and interpersonal stigma. Lack of social safety exacerbates the chronic threat vigilance of minority stress and compounds the negative long-term effects on cognitive, emotional, and immunologic functioning.[13,14] Many LGBTQ+ individuals may have both minority stress and lack of social safety creating cumulative effects in their experience with serious illness. Taking a patient-centered approach, palliative care teams view the person beyond the disease and can help address social safety concerns, improve their quality of life, and empower families of choice.

Recommendations

In order to best serve LGBTQ+ older adults, the authors recommend a trauma-informed care approach and better understanding the biases in end-of-life care.

Trauma-Informed Care

Trauma-informed care is an organizational approach to care that assumes that everyone who encounters the system might have had a past traumatic event. The goal is to enact practices to avoid retraumatization.[15] This approach is critical in palliative and end-of-life care because past trauma plays a role in how people react to and cope with pain, serious illness, change in function, and loss.

Utilizing the ADDRESSING model in **Table 1**, clinicians can explore individualistic life experiences that might contribute to trauma including childhood and adult physical abuse, emotional abuse, sexual abuse, neglect, intimate partner violence, and community violence, as well as structural violence in our society including racism, sexism, xenophobia, homophobia, and transphobia.

Maladaptive responses to trauma experiences that lie dormant for long periods may emerge later in life or when facing serious diseases. The possibility of death itself is a trauma and a history of psychological trauma can make managing the symptoms of end of life more challenging. This challenge arises from the association of trauma history with post-traumatic stress disorder (PTSD) and higher levels of chronic pain. Also, life review is a common practice that focuses on meaning-making and closure among people who are dying, and this may include the integration of past traumatic events which may retraumatize the individual. Prior trauma can also resurface in family members or even the care team. For palliative care and hospice providers, such experiences may be particularly difficult due to repeated exposure to death and reactivation of prior trauma.

Clinical Pearl: Look for Markers of Trauma

- Certain conditions that are highly correlated with recent and past trauma include heart, lung, and liver diseases; obesity and diabetes; substance abuse and overdose; and mental health issues such as depression, PTSD, and anxiety.
- If these are on a patient's problem list, consider screening further for a history of trauma.

Trauma-informed care can help mitigate disparities and create a space of safety and support. For LGBTQ+ older adults, histories of trauma, including minority stress/discrimination and adverse childhood events, are strongly associated with future burden of physical and mental illnesses. This means that past or present trauma may be an active factor in decision-making for any patient facing a serious illness and more so when the serious illness is combined with other societal experiences as in LGBTQ+ older adults.

Several evidence-based approaches to trauma-informed care have been developed. An important element in all of these approaches is the initial screening for histories of trauma, which ideally should be done as early as possible. Universal screening reduces the risk of providers making assumptions about burdens of trauma merely because of a patient's racial, ethnic, and/or sexual identity.

For palliative care, the authors recommend using the 5 principles of trauma-informed care that include providing safety, establishing trust, enabling patient choice, facilitating collaboration, and empowering the patient. Utilizing the framework of trauma-informed care, there has been an important shift from considering "what is wrong with you?" which can trigger past trauma or lead to shame to "what has happened to you and how can our team best support you and your family of choice?" Open-ended, nonjudgmental questions in a safe, affirming clinical space can prove crucial in learning about a patient's trauma history. To set this stage, one might share, "Difficult life experiences, like growing up in a family where you were hurt, or where there was mental illness or drug/alcohol issues, or witnessing violence, can affect our health. Do you feel like any of your past experiences affect your physical or emotional health?" After experiences are shared, make sure to support the patient and acknowledge the bravery of sharing.

For palliative medicine patients experiencing progressive and serious illnesses on top of normal aging, an awareness of the presence of psychological trauma is important. Traumatic events including engagement in the health system (ie, ICU, hospital, clinic), interpersonal and intrapersonal stigma (ie,internalized homophobia), historical events (ie,the AIDS epidemic and survivorship), and other serious illness end-of-life experiences can compound the expression and experience of total pain (ie,physical, psychological, social and spiritual) and symptom burden. This reality highlights the importance of adopting affirming care, since these elements of someone's health may be unknown and unaddressed unless they are screened (see N.M. Javier & R. Noy's, "Affirming Care for LGBTQ+ Patients", in this issue).

Recognizing Bias and Earning Trust

Trust is the cornerstone of a successful clinical relationship with a patient facing a serious illness. Yet stigma and the multitude of isms and phobias (ageism, racism, transphobia, homophobia) are ubiquitous within society as well as within medical institutions. These forms of historical and present discrimination perpetuate health disparities and contribute to worse health outcomes.[16,17] As discussed earlier, this is especially true for sexual and gender minority people and bias can show up and create barriers to care. The SEEDS model describes different forms of bias that might show up in palliative or end-of life care, including 1) similarity bias where people have differential responses to people who are more similar to them, 2) expedience or confirmation bias such as a lack of openness to hearing from something from a patient that goes against what the provider expects or believes, 3) experience bias where people may project their own assumptions about quality of life on their patients or may assume they know about the patient because of past interactions with similar patients, 4) distance bias where priority may be given to the most vocal family member over what has been documented about a patient's longstanding values, 5) safety bias such as favoring choices based on risk aversion or sunk cost, or based on misleading way of framing (eg, "Should we do everything for your loved one or should we switch to comfort care?").[18–22]

Being aware of bias, the presence of microaggressions, and the impact of verbal and nonverbal language is essential. This is especially true when an individual is confronted with a serious illness, letting us view their coping through the lens of minority stress and social safety. A nonjudgmental, culturally humble approach is recommended to best support the individual being cared for at the intersection of their identities and their illness.

Approach Decision-Making with Cultural Humility

What are the specific ways in which specific LGBTQ+ cultural identities inform decision-making at the end of life? Because there is no one-to-one correspondence between cultural identity and decision-making style, here the authors will highlight the patterns of decision-making themselves. These are some of the main questions and possibilities to assess with each individual patient and family.

First, who makes the medical decisions? In Western bioethics and legal systems, if a patient has mental capacity and legal competence to make medical decisions, that is their unassailable right. Yet patients of different cultures choose to involve families of choice or community in their decision-making to a lesser or greater extent. Studies have shown that the majority of participants across all demographic groups preferred an approach of shared decision-making.[20]

Second, how much information should be disclosed to the patient? Once again, Western bioethics and legal systems have 1 clear approach: it is the patient's right to know everything. Yet some patients will prefer **not** to know all their diagnostic and prognostic information, and that is also their right. In some communities, there is a belief that bad news or discussing death will hasten death.[21]

Third, what are the health disparities and associated barriers to care? How can they be addressed? As cited earlier in the article, challenges with access to care, acceptance, and stigma can create barriers seen more commonly in LGBTQ+ communities.

Fourth, what are the meanings ascribed to suffering, to dignity, and to death? How do these differing meanings translate into differing priorities for end-of-life treatments and trajectories? What takes priority: struggle or comfort?

In sum, these domains of difference give a sense of the great heterogeneity both across and within the LGBTQ+ community. The clinician must, therefore, adopt an open and nonjudgmental approach to respond appropriately to the cultural nuances in the decision-making process and help create a patient-centered care plan.

To reduce bias and stigma, the authors recommend incorporating standardized assessments of such preferences into the care of every patient, instead of attempting to guess when particular patients or families of choice might have divergent perspectives. In **Box 2**, the authors describe best practices for addressing LGBTQ+-inclusive decision-making or advance care planning.

DISCUSSION

The authors emphasize that any clinician, not just those working in palliative care, can and should use an approach to shared decision-making that is informed by cultural humility and structural competency.

Communication in serious illnesses and end-of-life care should be regarded as a procedure that improves with practice and a standardized, patient-centered approach. Studies show that patients wish to speak with clinicians frankly to receive

Box 2
Recommendations for addressing decision-making in serious illness

1. Adapt existing best practices around value-based, shared decision-making to mitigate bias and foster person-centered care.
   a. Resources: Prepare For Your Care (https://prepareforyourcare.org/), ACP videos (https://acpdecisions.org), Respecting Choices (https://respectingchoices.org), Vital Talk (https://vitaltalk.org).
   b. Techniques: Scripting, using in-person interpreters in settings of language nonconcordance, drawing on cultural brokers within the health system or from the patient's community.
2. Clarify the different types of decision-making to the patient.
   a. Include the family members of choice to the degree that the patient desires.
3. Acknowledge mistrust and stigma in the health care system.
   a. Ask open-ended questions to determine whether the patient has experienced discrimination or breaches of trust from any past or current providers.
4. Evaluate, acknowledge, and make strategies to address social determinants of health and barriers to care, including but not limited to
   a. Transportation options
   b. Insurance needs
   c. Documented versus undocumented status

as much information as possible and to feel that they have been heard as people rather than patients. Yet clinicians use medical jargon, fail to recognize that the patient or family is not following, miss cues that patients are experiencing emotions that affect information absorption, or block patient questions and concerns. The result is divergence in illness understanding between what physicians believe they have communicated and what patients believe they have heard.[22]

There are numerous evidence-based approaches to communicating with patients with serious illnesses to achieve goal-concordant care. In this article, the authors will refer to the SUPER³ model created by the Clinician Patient Communication and Life Care Planning group of the Southern California Permanente Medical Group (**Fig. 1**). This model incorporates ADDRESSING intersectionality, evaluating bias, and trauma-informed care (Refer **Box 3** for how to use the model).

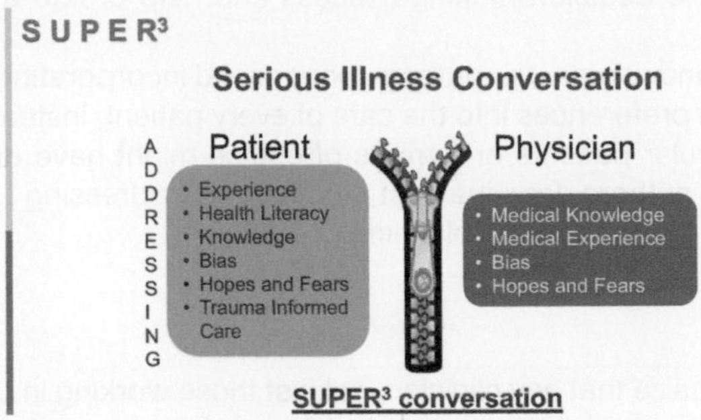

Fig. 1. The SUPER³ model (*Adapted from* the original content developed by the Southern California Permanente Medical Group Life Care Planning Program)

Box 3
Sample scripting using the SUPER³ model

1. Setup
   a. Assess decision makers, awareness of clinical circumstance, and evaluation of family:
      i. "Who is someone you trust to make decisions for you if you are very sick?"
      ii. "I'd like to talk about some decisions that people with your health conditions often face—is that OK?"
      iii. "How are health care decisions made in your family or support system?"
   b. Ensure shared understanding of the decision maker role:
      i. A person who knows your values, wishes, and what is important to you.
      ii. A person who agrees to be your decision maker.
      iii. A person who is able to make decisions in difficult situations
      iv. A person who agrees to follow your wishes even if different from their own
2. Understanding
   a. Assess patient's or decision maker's understanding of the situation and address gaps:
      i. "What do you understand about your illness?"
      ii. "What have the doctors told you about that?"
      iii. "Do you feel that you have a good understanding of what to expect over time?"
3. Past experiences
   a. Assess prior hospitalizations, prior treatments, and context and experience with the condition (eg, family members who went through a similar illness):
      i. "Do you know anyone else with this condition?"
      ii. "What did you learn from your last treatment? Last hospital stay?"
      iii. "Have you had experiences with family members who were very sick? Family members who were in the ICU? Who were on life support?"

4. Elicit values
   a. Assess personal goals, spiritual/religious affiliation, and other cultural influences:
      i. "What abilities matter so much to you that you can't imagine living without them?"
      ii. "What do you look forward to each day?"
      iii. "What does quality of life (living well) mean for you?"
      iv. "Do you have spiritual or religious beliefs that might inform your medical decisions?"
5. Review/Recommend/Record (R3)
   a. Review—recap the discussion to ensure agreement. You may need to provide additional information to bridge any misunderstanding.
      i. "It sounds like..."
      ii. "What I heard was..."
   b. Recommend—seek to align patient's goals and values with the treatment options being offered, asking permission to provide your own clinical recommendation:
      i. "Based on what we know about your health condition, and what I heard you say is important, I have some recommendations. Would that be OK?"
      ii. If the patient's values lead you to recommend do-not-resuscitate (DNR) status:
         1. "I recommend a natural dying process. We'll make sure to prioritize your comfort and support your children. In medical language, this is a DNR order."
         2. "I wish intubation and tube feeding would cure the underlying ________."
      iii. "If you were to receive _______ what would you expect?"
      iv. "What concerns, if any, do you have about making this decision?"
   c. Record—make note of the information you have learned in the discussion somewhere it will be easily accessible. It is essential to document any changes for treatment course or code status.
6. Repeat as many times as necessary, as the disease and the situation evolve.

SUMMARY

Palliative care focuses on improving the quality of life for people with serious illnesses and their loved ones. This article introduces considerations including barriers to care, intersectionality, minority stress, microaggressions, and social safety that may impact the experience and openness of people to receive this care. The authors outline tools to address these challenges including trauma-informed care and how to recognize bias and earn trust. The authors conclude by offering a model for incorporating these assessments and tools with sample scripts to provide patient-centered and holistic palliative care. Though this article focuses on palliative and hospice care for LGBTQ+ patients, the themes and tools can be extended to a broader patient population to provide high-quality and inclusive palliative care. When possible, the authors recommend connecting LGBTQ+ patients with teams and resources known to support the LGBTQ+ community. The use of out lists or tips for finding LGBTQ+ affirming care (https://www.lgbtagingcenter.org/resources/resource.cfm?r=4) can help to ensure appropriate and sensitive care for serious illnesses, end-of-life, and postmortem planning and care.

Further Learning

The authors recommend the following resources for people and organizations wishing to improve the quality of palliative and hospice care provided to LGBTQ+ people:

- Acquaviva, Kimberly D., "LGBTQ-Inclusive Hospice and Palliative Care: A Practical Guide to Transforming Professional Practice" (2017). *Faculty Bookshelf*. 107. https://hsrc.himmelfarb.gwu.edu/books/107

- Maingi S, Bagabag AE, O'Mahony S. Current Best Practices for Sexual and Gender Minorities in Hospice and Palliative Care Settings. J Pain Symptom Manage. 2018 May;55(5):1420-1427. https://doi.org/10.1016/j.jpainsymman.2017.12.479. Epub 2017 Dec 27. PMID: 29288882

ACKNOWLEDGMENTS

The authors would like to thank Masil George for her contributions to the article.

DISCLOSURE

The authors have no disclosures.

REFERENCES

1. Acquaviva K. LGBTQ-inclusive hospice and palliative medicine: a practical Guide to transforming professional practice. New York, NY: Harrington Park Press; 2017.
2. Quill TE, Abernethy AP. Generalist plus specialist palliative care–creating a more sustainable model. N Engl J Med 2013;368(13):1173–5.
3. Berkman C, Stein GL, Godfrey D, et al. Disrespectful and inadequate palliative care to lesbian, gay, and bisexual patients. Palliat Support Care 2023;1–6. https://doi.org/10.1017/S1478951523001037. Published online July 12.
4. Berkman C, Stein GL, Javier NM, et al. Disrespectful and inadequate palliative care to transgender persons. Palliat Support Care 2023;1–7. https://doi.org/10.1017/S1478951523001104. Published online July 14.
5. de Vries B. Persons in the second half of life: the intersectional influences of stigma and cohort. LGBT Health 2014;1(1):18–23.
6. de Vries B, Mason AM, Quam J, et al. State recognition of same-sex relationships and preparations for end of life among lesbian and gay boomers. Sex Res Soc Policy 2009;6(1):90–101.
7. Kemery SA. Family perceptions of quality of end of life in LGBTQ+ individuals: a comparative study. Palliat Care Soc Pract 2021;15. https://doi.org/10.1177/26323524211997153. 26323524211997153.
8. Hays P. Addressing cultural complexities in practice: assessment, diagnosis and therapy. American Psychological Association; 2008.
9. Clark K, Phillips J. End of life care - the importance of culture and ethnicity. Aust Fam Physician 2010;39(4):210–3.
10. Meyer IH. Prejudice, social stress, and mental health in lesbian, gay, and bisexual populations: conceptual issues and research evidence. Psychol Bull 2003;129(5):674–97.
11. Sue DW, Capodilupo CM, Torino GC, et al. Racial microaggressions in everyday life: implications for clinical practice. Am Psychol 2007;62(4):271–86.
12. Nadal KL, Whitman CN, Davis LS, et al. Microaggressions toward lesbian, gay, bisexual, transgender, queer, and genderqueer people: a review of the literature. J Sex Res 2016;53(4–5):488–508.
13. Diamond LM, Alley J. Rethinking minority stress: a social safety perspective on the health effects of stigma in sexually-diverse and gender-diverse populations. Neurosci Biobehav Rev 2022;138:104720.
14. American Psychiatric Association. Diagnostic and Statistical Manual of Mental Disorders. 5th ed.; 2013.

15. Harris M, Fallot R. Using trauma theory to design service systems. Jossey-Bass; 2001.
16. Institute of Medicine (US) committee on understanding and eliminating racial and ethnic disparities in health care. In: Smedley BD, Stith AY, Nelson AR, editors. Unequal treatment: confronting racial and ethnic disparities in health care. National Academies Press (US); 2003. Available at: http://www.ncbi.nlm.nih.gov/books/NBK220358/. Accessed August 30, 2023.
17. Spencer K, Grace M. Social foundations of health care inequality and treatment bias | annual review of sociology. Annu Rev Sociol 2016;42:101–20.
18. Lieberman MD, Rock D, Halvorson HG, Cox C. Breaking bias updated: The seeds model. Neuroleadership J 2015;6:4–18.
19. Kripke C. Patients with disabilities: avoiding unconscious bias when discussing goals of care. Am Fam Physician 2017;96(3):192–5.
20. Chiu C, Feuz MA, McMahan RD, et al. "Doctor, make my decisions": decision control preferences, advance care planning, and satisfaction with communication among diverse older adults. J Pain Symptom Manag 2016;51(1):33–40.
21. Colclough YY, Brown GM. End-of-life treatment decision making: American Indians' perspective. Am J Hosp Palliat Care 2014;31(5):503–12.
22. Back AL, Fromme EK, Meier DE. Training clinicians with communication skills needed to match medical treatments to patient values. J Am Geriatr Soc 2019; 67(S2):S435–41.

Home-Based Care for Lesbian, Gay, Bisexual, Transgender, Queer or Questioning, or another diverse gender identity Older Adults

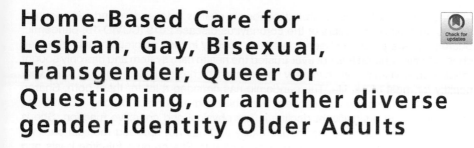

Mariah L. Robertson, MD, MPH

KEYWORDS

• Hospital-at-home • Home-based medical care • Home care • Homebound
• Trauma-informed care • Health disparities • LGBTQ+

KEY POINTS

- Home-based medical care is rapidly expanding to meet the ever-growing needs of homebound older adults, the highest risk and highest cost patients in the health care system.
- Little is currently understood about the prevalence of lesbian, gay, bisexual, transgender, queer or questioning, or another diverse gender identity (LGBTQ+) homebound older adults, but given what we understand about the epidemiology of both groups, we can postulate a significant overlap exists.
- To provide patient-centered and trauma-informed care of LGBTQ+ older adults at home, clinicians and home-based care teams must take a thoughtful, evidence-based, and universal approach to providing inclusive and affirming care.
- It is paramount that home-based care organizations and health systems utilize existing resources to provide universal training for all care providers and interdisciplinary team members to ensure inclusive, patient-centered, and affirming care is prioritized for all older adults at home.
- Future efforts in research should focus on understanding the intersectionality that exists within homebound older adults with a specific interest in understanding unique needs that exist for our LGBTQ+ homebound older adults.

Clinical vignette, Part 1

Sharon (she/her) is a 79-year-old cisgender lesbian woman who lives with her partner, Margaret (she/her), an 84-year-old transgender lesbian woman. They have been

Division of Geriatric Medicine and Gerontology, Department of Internal Medicine, Johns Hopkins School of Medicine, 5200 Eastern Avenue, Mason F. Lord Building/Center Tower/Ste 2200, Baltimore, MD 21224, USA
E-mail address: mdewsna1@jhmi.edu

Clin Geriatr Med 40 (2024) 347–356
https://doi.org/10.1016/j.cger.2023.10.006

together for over 20 years. Sharon describes herself as independent and self-assured, and up until the past 3 years of the coronavirus disease 2019 (COVID-19) pandemic, Sharon and Margaret had been very active socially in their community and with their chosen family. Sharon has not ever trusted the health care system and has only sought medical care when it was absolutely necessary. She has considered herself to be very healthy for most of her life. The pandemic has changed a lot for them both. Sharon caught COVID before vaccines were available, and as a result of long COVID, she has experienced a significant decline in her physical and cognitive function. She is now not able to get out of her house easily and has not received medical care for over 2 years. Margaret has been providing care to Sharon on a full-time basis and has been relying on spotty paid caregiver services to help when they can. Recently, Sharon was admitted to the hospital for a pulmonary embolism and on discharge the hospital social worker gave Margaret information on a new, home-based primary care program that Sharon would qualify for. Margaret is concerned about the new medications that Sharon needs and the complexity of her care already. She agrees to enroll Sharon in primary care at home, though she remains nervous about what this will be like.

INTRODUCTION

Home-based medical care is a rapidly expanding health care delivery ecosystem.[1] This is due to many factors including the inherent gaps in access to medical care in traditional, hospital-based medical settings, particularly for frail older adults living with multiple chronic conditions and physical debility. While many people harken back to times of "old-school" house calls, home-based medical care of the current

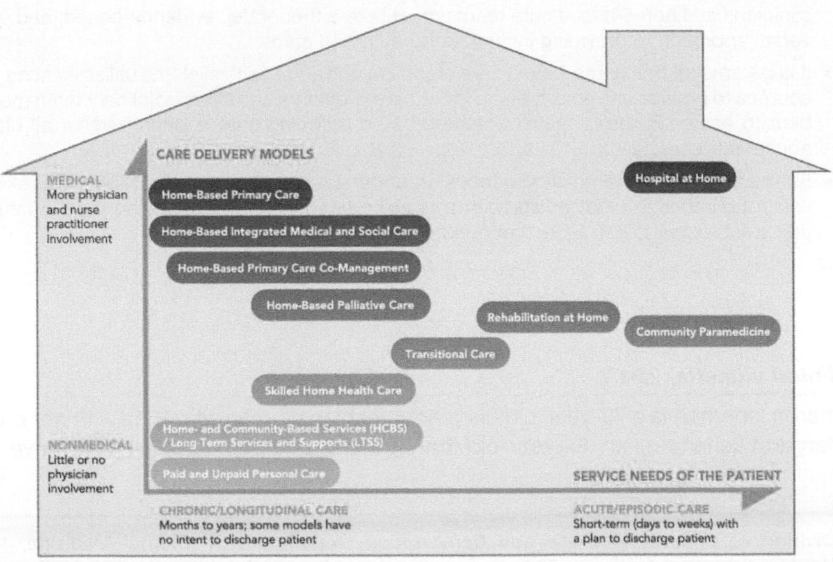

Notes: The relative size of the model labels does not reflect the numbers of patients served by or practices/systems using the model. *Community Paramedicine* refers to Mobile Integrated Health-Community Paramedicine.

Fig. 1. The landscape of home-based care*. (*From*: Ritchie C, Leff B, Gallopyn N, Pu C, Sheehan O. Medical care at home comes of age. 2021 Jan. *Reprinted with permission from the California Health care Foundation 2023.)

times is comprehensive in nature and encompasses everything from paid and unpaid personal care (eg, home health aides) all the way to hospital-level care at home and everything in between (**Fig. 1**). We are at a tipping point in health care delivery for our aging population. With the baby boom and rising numbers of older adults requiring health care, the health care system is shifting models of care delivery for more complex patients. As such we are seeing a change from volume-based to value based models of care delivery that focus on the quality of care and prevention of unnecessary health care utilization. This expansion has coincided with the COVID-19 pandemic, where we saw a doubling of homebound older adults, with the highest increase in populations at highest risk for health disparities due to social and structural factors. Specifically, we saw increases in homebound status among Black (9%–22%) and Hispanic/Latine (16.7%–34.5%) communities and communities with lower educational attainment and fewer financial resources or supports.[2] During the pandemic, we have also seen rapid innovations in the space of virtual and telemedicine care and allocation of Medicare funding for hospital-at-home for the first time, an innovation that was decades in the making.[3–5]

In many important ways, expansion of home-based medical care improves inherent inequities in access to medical care. By meeting patients where they are, we are eliminating some of the key barriers to care that exist for marginalized and minoritized populations. However, with any rapidly expanding models of care delivery, we must be thoughtful about the inclusivity of the care we are providing. This is especially true for our lesbian, gay, bisexual, transgender, queer or questioning, or another diverse gender identity (LGBTQ+) homebound older adults.[6] It is the goal of this article to discuss how home-based care providers can be more thoughtful about the care of homebound LGBTQ+ older adults.

DEFINITIONS AND CONNECTIONS

For this article, we define homebound as someone living in the community but rarely or never leaving the home in the prior month.[2] We define intersectionality as the ways in which systems of inequality based on gender, race, ethnicity, sexual orientation, gender identity, physical ability, class, and other forms of discrimination intersect to impact health and social experiences.[7–9] For many years the homebound population has not been well studied or understood. As such, it has been difficult to elucidate the specific disparities that exist within this population. In recent years, more epidemiologic data have been published and we are better able to understand the existing inequities. Specifically, homebound older adults are more likely to be single, nonwhite, financially impoverished, and socially isolated.[10] The intersectionality of these factors increases the risk that homebound older adults have had prior, cumulative traumas in their lives and increases their risk for poorer health outcomes.

There are currently at least 3 million LGBTQ+ adults over the age of 50 in the United States and that is projected to increase to more than 7 million by 2030.[11] Traditional health care spaces have not always felt safe for LGBTQ+ older adults. More than 80% of LGBTQ+ older adults have experienced 1 or more instance of victimization or discrimination in health care settings in their lifetime.[12] Additionally, seeking senior housing and long-term care for LGBTQ+ older adults is wrought with discrimination and potential trauma. In fact, nearly half (48%) of same-sex couples have reported adverse treatment when searching for senior housing and more than half of states (29) lack inclusion of sexual orientation or gender identity in housing protections for older adults.[11,13] LGBTQ+ older adults experience very similar health disparities to homebound older adults. In fact, LGBTQ+ older adults are twice as likely to be single and live alone and 4 times less likely to have adult children when compared to their straight, cisgender peers.[14] LGBTQ+ older adults are more likely to experience poverty and social isolation. In fact, over half (59%) of LGBTQ+ older adults lack companionship and 53% feel isolated from others. Many LGBTQ+ older adults may both need long-term care and be reluctant to enter it for fear of discrimination and lack of housing protection.[15] In similar ways as seen in our homebound older adults, the COVID-19 pandemic has shown increased rates of poverty, depression, and anxiety, with twice as many reporting a lack of access to adequate mental health services when compared to their straight, cisgender peers.[16]

While to the author's knowledge, there currently exist no published data specifically evaluating the health outcomes of homebound LGBTQ+ older adults, the above data and overlap in disparities in these populations suggest a significant need for both epidemiologic research in this space and discussion on training for the home-care workforce in inclusive, trauma-informed care (TIC) of this population.

Clinical Vignette, Part 2: Planning for the Visit

Sharon and Margaret are nervous about a home-based primary care team coming out to their home. When they received the intake call, Margaret was veiled in her description of their relationship. She told the team she was Sharon's best friend and caregiver. Sharon has some memory changes that make explaining the nature of the visit at home a bit complicated, but Margaret has taken the time to explain it to Sharon a few times. Margaret knows that ever since her mother died at a very young age from cancer, Sharon has not trusted doctors. Sharon feels certain her mother was treated differently because of her race. This fear of health care has been further amplified by the way in which they have seen friends in the LGBTQ+ community treated by health care workers in the past. Between the human immunodeficiency virus epidemic and many friends going back into the closet for long-term care services, they have seen a lot of harm come to people they love at the hands of health care systems. They are nervous about letting anyone into their home, which has been their safe haven from many things they have faced in their life. Margaret is especially afraid that now that they are both aging and Sharon is so frail, the health care team will force them to go into a nursing home.

CARING FOR LESBIAN, GAY, BISEXUAL, TRANSGENDER, QUEER OR QUESTIONING, OR ANOTHER DIVERSE GENDER IDENTITY OLDER ADULTS AT HOME

In home-based medical care, we view our work as both patient-centered and focused on health equity. Home-based care teams are meeting people where they are, in their home environments, and eliminating many of the barriers that exist to accessing care in more traditional ways.[6] That said, it is important to note that the home might be the safest of safe spaces for our patients, particularly LGBTQ+ older adults. Many fear "returning to the closet" if they require nursing home care for any reason, the same fear may also be true (and potentially amplified) in home-based medical care.[15] The idea of health care providers coming into the home might be traumatizing or retraumatizing for our patients, particularly on a first visit. As such, it is paramount that we are approaching the home with adequate training in trauma-informed and inclusive care.

There are many models to consider when thinking about the most inclusive, patient-centered ways to approach a visit to our patient's home. For this article we will draw from 2 models that are both important to inclusive and thoughtful care of patients, the Substance Abuse and Mental Health Services Administration's 6 principles of TIC[17] and the Stanford Presence 5.[18–20] Neither model is specifically designed for home-based care of LGBTQ+ populations; however, both are validated in populations who are often victimized, minoritized, and marginalized by health care systems and both approach providing care in a 'universal precautions' way.[18,21,22] This means working to suspend assumptions and approaching every patient in an inclusive, thoughtful, patient-centered, and trauma-informed manner. **Table 1** gives a framework for approaching a home visit and ties this approach to the core components of these 2 models.

With the current rapid expansion of programs like hospital-at-home and home-based primary care, there is a breadth of individuals entering the home environment including physicians (eg, family and internal medicine, geriatric medicine, hospice, and palliative care); advanced practice providers; nurses; physical, occupational, and speech therapists; social workers; community health workers; and home health aides, among others. This framework, while focused on the clinician's approach to a home visit, will hopefully be applicable, in part, to the many facets of home-based care.

Clinical Vignette, Part 3: the Home Visit

Dr. James, the clinician who came out to visit Sharon and Margaret at home, had received training in TIC and had undergone specific additional training in the care of LGBTQ+ older adults—enough so that she was listed on the LGBTQ+ Health care Directory.[23] Dr. James greeted Sharon and Margaret at the door and was wearing a pin that signaled both that she was an ally and her pronouns (she/her). Upon entering the home and sitting down to chat, her first question was what pronouns both Sharon and Margaret used. These initial signs were such an overwhelming relief for them both; they could feel themselves relaxing into the visit. It was clear that Dr. James' goal was to be there for and supportive of Sharon and Margaret. This meant being curious and thoughtful about what matters most to Sharon and Margaret and asking important questions about their chosen family. This also meant allowing Margaret to lead and assuring her that she could end the visit at any time. Dr. James centered the age-friendly 4 M's (medications, mentation, matters most, mobility)[24] but did so in a way that was inclusive and thoughtful. She also asked about sexual orientation and gender identity in an unassuming and thoughtful way that made both Sharon and Margaret feel seen and heard and not judged. Toward the end of the visit, Dr. James offered Margaret enrollment in their program as well, acknowledging the important and often unseen role of a caregiver of homebound older adults. Margaret had been neglecting her own health for some time and agreed that Dr. James might just be the right person to help her get back on track with screening and other important health care tasks. They worked together to set an agenda for the next visit and Sharon, despite undergoing some questions about memory and health, was open to continuing to be seen and treated by the home-based medicine team. Dr. James enlisted the help of her social work and community health colleagues to help connect Sharon and Margaret to community resources including meals on wheels and home health as well as some key community resources for LGBTQ+ older adults. They planned to connect again in 1 month.

FUTURE DIRECTIONS AND RESOURCES FOR ORGANIZATIONS AND HEALTH SYSTEMS

While we have begun the discussion in this article with some thoughts about how we can better approach home visits as clinicians with our LGBTQ+ older adult patients in mind, with a clinical vignette to provide examples of care, this is just the beginning of the discussion. Each clinician exists within an organization, each organization within

Table 1
Approaching a home visit with lesbian, gay, bisexual, transgender, queer or questioning, or another diverse gender identity older adults

Components of Visit	Inclusive Ways to Approach the Visit	Trauma-Informed Care Principles	Presence 5 Principles
Pre-visit preparation	Ensure you signal inclusivity where you can: for example, pride pins, pronouns.	Safety Trustworthiness & transparency	Prepare with intention
	Pre-visit call: use pronouns, ask theirs, ensure important people will be present if they prefer, and ensure comfort with the visit.	Safety Trustworthiness & transparency Empowerment, voice, & choice	
	Pre-chart: familiarize yourself with the patient you are meeting, their support system/chosen family, and important details of their story.	Cultural, historical, & gender issues	
Start of visit	Introduce self with pronouns, ask for theirs, and ensure everyone in the room is identified and acknowledged.	Safety Trustworthiness & transparency	Listen intently & completely
	Signal safety: minimize incursion on space, sit at level of the patient, center the patient when talking, and proceed according to the patient's comfort with the visit/exam/questions.		
	Collaboratively identify an agenda for the visit that centers the patient's concerns.	Collaboration & mutuality Empowerment, voice, & choice	
	Ensure amplification device and other sensory assistive devices are present so the patient can completely participate. Minimize external distractions where possible.	Trustworthiness & transparency	
	Use language that is inclusive always and does not assume gender identity or sexual orientation of anyone until more history has been taken and relationships understood.	Cultural, historical, & gender issues	

Mid-visit: a focus on geriatric and home-based skills	Engagement with chosen family and support system. Assess for burden/burnout.	Collaboration & mutuality	Listens intently & completely
	Actively listen to patient • Review medications. • Examine mobility and function. • Screen for mentation changes (eg, depression, dementia, delirium) • Ask appropriate SOGI questions if first visit. • Discuss goals and what matters most to them including organ-specific screening tests where appropriate. • Celebrate efforts and successes!	Trustworthiness & transparency Empowerment, voice, & choice	Listens intently & completely Connect with the patient's story Explore emotional cues
	Assure patient and caregivers they can end the visit at any time if they are uncomfortable. Validate emotions as they arise.	Safety Empowerment, voice, & choice Cultural, historical, & gender issues	Explore emotional cues
Visit closure: closing the loop and planning for appropriate follow-up	Care plan including testing is made in collaboration with the patient, chosen family, and what matters most. Teach back for understanding.	Collaboration & mutuality	Agree on what matters most Explore emotional cues
	Where appropriate, ensure documentation is in place for end-of-life planning that includes partners/caregivers (eg, advance directives).	Empowerment, voice & choice Cultural, historical & gender issues	Connect with the patient's story
	Consider connecting to peer support groups for social support, including virtual and telephone-based supports where possible through organizations such as SAGE.	Cultural, historical, & gender issues	

Abbreviations: SAGE, Services and Advocacy for Lesbian, Gay, Bisexual, and Transgender Elders; SOGI, sexual orientation and gender identity.

a health system, and each health system within a governmental structure that does not yet fully value home-based models of care or the patients they serve. The battle ahead is large.

While policies and governmental structures take time to shift, it remains paramount that the organizations that deliver home-based care services start to change now. This means employing expertise from existing organizations such as Services and Advocacy for LGBT Elders (SAGE) and their National Resource Center for LGBTQ+ Aging, who has been doing this work for decades. SAGECare, an educational resource for LGBTQ+ aging cultural competency, has worked to develop training programs and strategic guidance for organizations and policy makers.[25] They have successfully assisted with state-required trainings in LGBTQ+ aging for long-term care and home health care teams in California, New York, and New Jersey. FORGE as an organization has existed since 1994 and has worked to reduce the impact of trauma on trans and non-binary survivors and communities through education, advocacy, and connection.[26] Fenway Health, a Boston-based health care organization that has been providing essential services to sexual and gender minority patients since the early 1970s, has also developed several trainings through the LGBTQIA + Aging Project which can be used by health systems and organizations to train their workforce.[27] These are just a few examples of ways we can support the work already being done to change systems of care for LGBTQ+ homebound older adults. There is much work to be done; honoring the existing allies and community members and paying them for the work they are doing will help ensure its reach is magnified.

SUMMARY

This article aims to educate the workforce caring for homebound LGBTQ+ older adults about the need to provide inclusive, affirming, and TIC. There are some specific recommendations and suggested frameworks for approaching a home visit as a clinician. We also provided a clinical vignette to show how using a patient-centered and trauma-informed approach to care of LGBTQ+ older adults can help ally and create inclusive spaces for care within the home. It is the author's hope that this approach can be applied across disciplines within home care medicine. But most importantly, a goal of this article is to raise awareness of existing resources and organizations that have been doing the important work of education, advocacy, and community support for decades now. It is our role as clinicians to continue to educate ourselves on how to provide care that creates safe spaces for our LGBTQ+ patients wherever the care is delivered, but particularly when it is delivered in the home.

CLINICS CARE POINTS

- Care at home provides an opportunity to eliminate barriers for patients at highest risk for disparities in access to care but it must be inclusive and trauma-informed.
- LGBTQ+ older adults are at risk for retraumatization when home-based care teams are entering the home without adequate training in affirming and inclusive care.
- Using existing frameworks and resources to help scaffold existing approaches to the care of LGBTQ+ older adults at home will help ensure that patients feel safe, supported, and heard by their home-based medical care teams.

DISCLOSURE

The author has no relevant financial disclosures.

FUNDING

The Author funded through HRSA grant number K01HP49050-01-00.

REFERENCES

1. Ritchie C, Leff B, Gallopyn N, et al. Medical care at home comes of age. Medical Care at Home Comes of Age 2021;1658–60.
2. Ankuda CK, Leff B, Ritchie CS, et al. Association of the COVID-19 pandemic with the prevalence of homebound older adults in the United States, 2011-2020. JAMA Intern Med 2021;181.
3. Levine DM, Ouchi K, Blanchfield B, et al. Hospital-level care at home for acutely ill adults. Ann Intern Med 2020;172(2):77.
4. Gaillard G, Russinoff I. Hospital at home: a change in the course of care. J Am Assoc Nurse Pract 2023;35(3):179–82.
5. Patel HY, West DJ. Hospital at home: an evolving model for comprehensive healthcare. Global Journal on Quality and Safety in Healthcare 2021;4(4):141–6.
6. Robertson ML, Carnahan JL, Streed CG. Caring for LGBTQ+ older adults at home. J Gen Intern Med 2023;38(6):1538–40.
7. Center for intersectional justice 2020 narrative report. Berlin: Center for Intersectional Justice; 2021.
8. Crenshaw K. Mapping the margins: intersectionality, identity politics, and violence against women of color. Stanford Law Rev 1991;43(6):1241.
9. Bauer GR, Churchill SM, Mahendran M, et al. Intersectionality in quantitative research: a systematic review of its emergence and applications of theory and methods. SSM Popul Health 2021;14:100798.
10. Ornstein KA, Leff B, Covinsky KE, et al. Epidemiology of the homebound population in the United States. JAMA Intern Med 2015;175(7):1180.
11. SAGE. Out and Visible: The Experiences of Lesbian, Gay, Bisexual and Transgender Older Adults, Ages 45-75. 2014.
12. Choi SK, Meyer HH. LGBT Aging: A Review of Research Findings, Needs, and Policy Implications. . Los Angeles; 2016.
13. The Equal Rights Center. Opening Doors: An Investigation of Barriers to Senior Housing for Same-Sex Couples. 2014.
14. SAGE. Improving the Lives of LGBT Older Adults. 2010.
15. Caceres BA, Travers J, Primiano JE, et al. Provider and LGBT Individuals' perspectives on LGBT##w. Gerontol 2020;60(3):e169–83.
16. The UCLA School of Law Williams Institute. LGBT Adults Aged 50 and Older in the US During the COVID-19 Pandemic. Los Angeles ; 2023.
17. Samhsa. SAMHSA's Concept of Trauma and Guidance for a Trauma-Informed Approach. 2014.
18. Shankar M, Henderson K, Garcia R, et al. Presence 5 for racial justice workshop: fostering dialogue across medical education to disrupt anti-black racism in clinical encounters. MedEdPORTAL 2022;18:11227.
19. Zulman DM, Verghese A. Virtual care, telemedicine visits, and real connection in the era of COVID-19. JAMA 2021;325(5):437.

20. Zulman DM, Haverfield MC, Shaw JG, et al. Practices to foster physician presence and connection with patients in the clinical encounter. JAMA 2020; 323(1):70.
21. Raja S, Hasnain M, Hoersch M, et al. Trauma informed care in medicine. Fam Community Health 2015 Jul;38(3):216–26.
22. National Resource Center on LGBTQ+ Aging. Person-centered. Trauma-informed Care of Transgender Older Adults 2023.
23. LGBTQ+ Healthcare Directory. https://lgbtqhealthcaredirectory.org/.
24. Mate KS, Berman A, Laderman M, et al. Creating age-friendly health systems – a vision for better care of older adults. Healthcare 2018;6(1):4–6.
25. SAGECare. https://sageusa.care/.
26. FORGE. https://forge-forward.org/.
27. LGBTQIA+ Aging Project. https://fenwayhealth.org/the-fenway-institute/lgbtqia-aging-project/training/.

Federal and State Policy Issues Affecting Lesbian, Gay, Bisexual, Transgender, and Queer Older Adults

Sean R. Cahill, PhD

KEYWORDS

• Sexual orientation • Gender identity • Elder services • LGBTQ+ • Long-term care • Nondiscrimination • Culturally competent care • Health equity

KEY POINTS

- Anti-lesbian, gay, bisexual, transgender, and queer (LGBTQ) + discrimination hurts people's health and is a barrier to accessing care.
- Four in five Americans support sexual orientation and gender identity (SOGI) nondiscrimination laws.
- LGBTQ + people experience health disparities.
- Collecting and using SOGI data can improve quality of care through clinical decision support, informing preventive screenings, and population health management.

INTRODUCTION

There are a number of key public policy issues affecting lesbian, gay, bisexual, transgender, and queer (LGBTQ) + older adults at the state and federal level. These include nondiscrimination laws and regulations to ensure access to health care and the socioeconomic resources required to thrive and be healthy. Other health policy issues include insurance access and coverage; efforts to promote culturally responsive and clinically competent care; behavioral health care needs; and elder services and policy that are responsive to the needs of LGBTQ + older adults and older people living with human immnodeficiency virus (HIV).

Sexual Orientation and Gender Identity Nondiscrimination Laws and Regulations

Unfortunately, even though 80% of Americans support sexual orientation and gender identity (SOGI) nondiscrimination,[1] nondiscrimination laws inclusive of sexual orientation have been a key battleground in the United States since the early 1970s.[2] SOGI

The Fenway Institute, 1340 Boylston Street, Boston, MA 02215, USA
E-mail address: scahill@fenwayhealth.org

Clin Geriatr Med 40 (2024) 357–366
https://doi.org/10.1016/j.cger.2023.10.007 geriatric.theclinics.com

nondiscrimination laws and regulations can help ensure access to health care and the socioeconomic resources required to thrive and be healthy. Such laws are needed because LGBTQ + people experience widespread social discrimination. According to a 2023 Center for American Progress report, more than 1in 3 LGBTQI+[a] Americans faced discrimination in the past year. More than 20% of LGBTQI + Americans report postponing or avoiding medical treatment due to discrimination.[3] Discrimination based on SOGI negatively affects the health of LGBTQ + people and functions as a barrier to care.[4] Discrimination in health care may cause sexual and gender minority patients to have higher rates of medical mistrust, which can constitute a barrier to accessing care.[5] Anti-LGBTQ + discrimination likely contributes to health disparities experienced by LGBTQ + people, such as higher rates of diabetes,[6] cardiovascular disease,[7,8] kidney disease,[9] cancer,[10] and HIV.[11,12]

The Biden-Harris Administration interprets federal sex discrimination laws, which are referenced in the 2010 Affordable Care Act (ACA), to prohibit sexual orientation and gender identity discrimination as well,[13] following the logic of US Supreme Court Justice Neil Gorsuch, who wrote for a 6 to 3 majority in the landmark *Bostock v. Clayton County, Georgia* case (2020) that "it is impossible to discriminate against a person for being homosexual or transgender without discriminating against that individual based on sex."[14(p. 9)] Because Section 1557 of the ACA references Title IX of the Education Amendments of 1972, which prohibits sex discrimination, the US Department of Health and Human Services (HHS) stated in May 2021 that SOGI discrimination in health care is prohibited by federal law.[15] The Office of Civil Rights at HHS is currently (late 2023) finalizing a regulation that will codify this.[16] A 2016 implementing regulation issued by HHS during the Obama-Biden Administration stated that discrimination on the basis of gender identity, including against nonbinary and intersex individuals, as well as some forms of sexual orientation discrimination, constitute sex stereotyping and are prohibited by federal law.[17] This rule was challenged in federal court and reversed by HHS during the Trump-Pence Administration,[13] 1 of many anti-LGBTQ + actions taken by President Donald Trump.[18] The prohibition of SOGI discrimination in health care was reinstated by President Joe Biden.[14]

Anti-LGBTQ + religious right organizations have consistently challenged SOGI nondiscrimination policies in court. A recent example is the 2023 *Braidwood v. Becerra* decision, in which a federal court in Texas struck down a key provision of the ACA requiring full insurance coverage of preventive health screenings and services, such as mammograms. The employer in the case objected to covering pre-exposure prophylaxis (PrEP) for HIV prevention due to opposition to homosexuality.[19] Religious refusal policies, which proliferated at the federal level under President Trump and have been adopted in many states,[20] allow for the refusal of health care and social services if the provider of the care or services objects to the identity or behavior of the patient based on religious or moral belief. Such policies represent a major threat to the ability of LGBTQ + people to access health care and social services, such as anti-poverty programs or substance use treatment. They also take the concept of religious freedom and turn it on its head. True religious freedom protects an individual's right to worship—or not—and harms no one. Religious refusal policies cause third party harm to LGBTQ + people and others who are refused health care and social services. As Douglas NeJaime and Reva Siegel point out in *The Yale Law Review*, these laws inflict

[a] This article generally uses the acronym LGBTQ+, but some research cited is about LGBT people, or LGBTQI + people. When the author uses acronyms other than "LGBTQ+" it is to accurately cite the research study to which the author is referring.

both material harm and dignitary harm—harms that exacerbate stigma and reduce social status—on other citizens.[21]

Congressional passage of a federal SOGI nondiscrimination law would preempt most court challenges to the policy. The Equality Act would prohibit SOGI discrimination in employment, housing, public accommodations (including health care), and credit. The US House of Representatives passed the Equality Act in 2019, but then Senate Majority Leader Mitch McConnell refused to allow a vote on the bill. In the wake of the 2020 US Supreme Court ruling in *Bostock*, many Republican elected officials expressed support for SOGI nondiscrimination laws[22] (as do 80% of the USpublic).[1] A supermajority of 60 votes is needed to override a likely filibuster under Senate rules.

Federal SOGI nondiscrimination regulations and laws are needed in part because many Americans live in states that don't have SOGI nondiscrimination in state law. In 22 states and 4 US territories, there are no state laws prohibiting discrimination on the basis of SOGI.[23] Furthermore, many states have passed laws restricting the rights of transgender people to access gender-affirming care. While most of these laws are focused on youth,[24] some prohibit adults from accessing gender-affirming care as well.[25]

In addition to passing SOGI nondiscrimination laws, it is important that attorneys general, civil rights offices, and law enforcement publicize the existence of such laws and enforce them to protect LGBTQ + people against discrimination. This will reduce the deleterious health effects of discrimination, and improve access to health care.

Poverty and Insurance Coverage

Partly as a result of widespread societal discrimination, LGBT people are more likely than heterosexual, cisgender people to live in poverty, with transgender people, bisexuals, and people of color experiencing the highest rates of poverty within the LGBT community.[26] While poverty rates declined in part due to federal assistance during the coronavirus disease 2019 (COVID-19) pandemic in 2021, LGBT disparities persisted. In 2021, 12% of straight cisgender Americans were poor, and 17% of LGBT Americans were poor. Some 20% of straight, cisgender people of color were poor, and 25% of LGBT people of color were poor in 2021. Among White people, 7% of straight cisgender people were poor, and 13% of LGBT people were poor.[27] In 2020, 34.8% of transgender people were poor, but this percentage dropped to 21.2% in 2021.[27]

There is evidence that LGBT people experience disproportionate economic hardship. The US Census Bureau's Household Pulse survey found that, during the first year and a half of the COVID-19 pandemic, LGBT people experienced twice the rate of food insecurity (14% vs 7%), higher job loss, and twice the rate of depression and anxiety as straight and cisgender people.[28] Older LGBTQ people may experience relatively higher rates of economic hardship. An analysis of Massachusetts Behavioral Risk Factor Surveillance System survey data from 2016 to 2018 found that, compared to straight and cisgender people age 50 to 75, LGBT people age 50 to 75 were more likely to rent and less likely to own their home, and were nearly 3 times as likely to report difficulty paying for housing or food in the past year.[29]

Lack of access to health insurance is a key correlate of health disparities and another indicator of socioeconomic disadvantage. Sexual minority women are less likely to have health insurance and a primary care provider than heterosexual women. An analysis of 2013 to 2015 National Health Interview Survey data found that lesbian and gay women were significantly less likely to have health insurance (80.7% of sexual minority women vs 85.2% of heterosexual women) and a usual primary care provider (79.6% of sexual minority women vs 84% of heterosexual women) compared to heterosexual women.[30] Striking racial/ethnic disparities in insurance coverage—with American Indians and Alaska Natives, Hispanics, and Black people less likely to be insured than White non-Hispanic and Asian Pacific Islander people[31]—also affect LGBTQ + people of color.

The Affordable Care Act dramatically reduced the uninsurance rate among LGBT people. Between June/September 2013 and December 2014/March 2015, the percentage of LGB adults without health insurance decreased from 21.7% to 11.1%, which is a larger decrease than in the non-LGB adult population.[32]

Expanded eligibility for Medicaid, a key element of the ACA, has been especially important for people living with HIV in the United States, most of whom are gay and bisexual men. In 2013, when the ACA's Medicaid expansion was implemented, just 17% of the estimated 1.2 million Americans living with HIV had private health insurance.[33] The US Centers for Disease Control and Prevention and the Kaiser Family Foundation estimate that the percentage of people living with HIV (PLWH) who lacked any kind of health insurance coverage was 22% in 2012 and dropped to 15% in 2014, following implementation of key elements of health care reform. The percentage of PLWH on Medicaid increased from 36% in 2012 to 42% in 2014.[34] The ACA, and Medicaid expansion in particular, have been very important to covering the health care costs and needs of PLWH. In 2023, 40% of people living with are on Medicaid, versus 15% of the general population.[35]

Culturally Responsive Health Care for LGBTQ + Patients

A number of initiatives have been undertaken by federal and state government agencies for many years to promote culturally responsive care for LGBTQ + patients. The National lesbian, gay, bisexual, transgender, queer, intersex, and asexual(LGBTQIA) + Health Education Center, a federally-funded project of the Fenway Institute, has trained health centers since 2011 in how to provide culturally responsive and affirming care to LGBTQ + patients.[36] Some 1400 health centers provide care to some 30 million patients in the United States[37] One key component of culturally responsive care is the collection and use of SOGI data to inform clinical decision support, preventive screenings, and population health management.[38] Since 2015 when SOGI was included in the Office of the National Coordinator of Health Information Technology's Meaningful Use Stage 3 Guidelines,[39] health IT regulations have promoted the collection and use of SOGI to improve quality of care.[40] The Bureau of Primary Health Care at the Health Services and Resources Administration has required the reporting of de-identified SOGI data on adult health center patients since 2016 to better understand and address health disparities.[38] Increasingly hospitals and private practices are collecting and using SOGI data to improve care for LGBTQ + patients.

Integration of behavioral health care with primary care is essential to ensure that all patients are screened for depression, substance use disorder, and other behavioral health issues. LGBTQ + older adults experience elevated rates of depression,[41] loneliness,[42] anxiety, and substance use disorder.[43] Older PLWH—most of whom in the United States are gay and bisexual men or transgender women—experience higher rates of loneliness,[42] social isolation,[44] and lack of social support.[45] Older gay and bisexual men living with HIV have a disproportionately higher likelihood of family rejection,[46] being single, and a lower likelihood of having children,[47] in part due to anti-gay and HIV stigma. Many older gay and bisexual men living with HIV lost partners, friends, and even entire friendship networks to the HIV/acquired immunodeficiency syndrome (AIDS) epidemic, especially before the advent of anti-retroviral therapy in 1996. Some long-term survivors with HIV, people diagnosed prior to 1996, experience survivor guilt.[48] Depression is now a leading cause of morbidity and mortality among older people living with HIV, exceeding even that caused by HIV.[49] Untreated depression correlates with poorer health outcomes among older PLWH.[50]

A dearth of culturally competent mental health providers coupled with insurance access barriers are 2 major issues preventing older LGBTQ + people and older PLWH from accessing behavioral health care.[51] Federal and state health agencies should fund fellowship and mentorship programs to ensure that health professionals are trained in the unique primary care and behavioral health care needs of older LGBTQ + people and older PLWH. Health agencies should support student loan forgiveness programs and other incentives to encourage training in LGBTQ + cultural competency for both the existing provider workforce and future health professionals. They should also take steps to increase insurance reimbursement and require that mental health providers accept public and private insurance.

LGBTQ + Affirming Elder Services

Social support and social network size are resiliency factors that protect against behavioral health burden in older LGBTQ + adults.[52] State departments on aging and Area Agencies on Aging (AAAs) should designate older LGBTQ + people and older PLWH as populations of greatest social need under the Older Americans Act (OAA) in order to provide culturally targeted services to them. Older LGBTQ + people and older PLWH have unique needs and experiences, and may be in greater need of formal elder services due to lower rates of parenting and being more likely to live alone. At the same time, they may be less likely to access these services due to fear of experiencing stigma and discrimination in elder services, either by age peers or by service providers themselves. Designating LGBTQ + older adults and older PLWH as populations of greatest social need under the Older Americans Act would encourage elder service providers to think more explicitly about how they are meeting the needs of these populations, and how they are ensuring that they can access affirming, culturally responsive services. This can help increase targeting funding for elder services for these populations, and explicit inclusion of them in state, city, and AAA elder service planning. Six states have passed legislation designating LGBT older adults as a population of greatest social need under the OAA: California, Illinois, Vermont, New York, Pennsylvania, and Virginia. Four states—New York, Illinois, California, and Vermont—and the District of Columbia have designated older PLWH as a population of greatest social need.[53]

The Administration for Community Living, an agency of the US Department of Health and Human Services that includes the Administration on Aging, is considering designating LGBTQI + older adults and older PLWH as populations of greatest social need under the Older Americans Act and requiring state aging departments to do so as well.[54] Such a move could dramatically improve access to culturally responsive elder services for these populations. Codifying these groups as populations of greatest need into federal regulation would go a long way toward ensuring that LGBTQI + older adults and older PLWH can access nondiscriminatory, affirming elder services to help them thrive and age in place, especially in states that lack SOGI nondiscrimination laws.

Many older LGBTQ + people need home care assistance to be able to age in their homes, but are afraid of experiencing discrimination at the hands of home care aides.[55] This is true of elder services more broadly, too. Many older PLWH, especially Long-Term Survivors living with HIV, live alone and have multiple conditions, including diabetes and blindness, that leave them essentially homebound. Home care assistance is absolutely essential to these individuals' ability to age in place. Many older PLWH experience health disparities need home care to support them with activities of daily living. Access to home care is needed now more than ever to help older PLWH age in place in community, including individuals under age 60. In Massachusetts, advocates are seeking to allow PLWH under age 60 to access home care.[56] At the request of the LGBT Aging Project, Massachusetts passed a law in 2018 requiring that all elder service workers be trained in LGBT aging issues within 12 months of starting their job.[57] Advocates in Massachusetts are also advocating for an LGBTQI + Long-Term Care Bill of Rights, which would explicitly articulate what SOGI nondiscrimination in housing and public accommodations means for LGBTQI + residents of rehab facilities, assisted living, long-term care, and nursing homes.[58] Massachusetts has a number of LGBTQ + elder policy innovations, including 2 dozen congregate meal programs for LGBTQ + elders and their friends funded with OAA funds, which are considered a national model.[59]

SUMMARY

Many older LGBTQ + people fought hard to win legal equality in the form of sexual orientation and gender identity nondiscrimination laws, marriage equality, nondiscrimination in immigration policy, military service, and in other areas. Many are now entering an elder service system that is not equipped to provide culturally responsive, nondiscriminatory care. While significant strides have been made over the past decade to improve culturally competent and affirming health care, an orchestrated political backlash against gender-affirming care for transgender people is undermining this progress. While there is strong societal support for marriage equality and SOGI nondiscrimination, some political leaders dismiss these equitable policies as "wokeness" and a threat to freedom of religion. LGBTQ + older adults experience health disparities, but these disparities can be reduced and even eliminated by collecting and using SOGI data to improve quality of care, and by advocating for an end to anti-LGBTQ + discrimination and stigma. SOGI nondiscrimination laws must be publicized and enforced, and elder services reformed, to ensure that LGBTQ + older adults can thrive and age in place.

DISCLOSURE

Fenway Health is a subrecipient of a grant to MPact: Global Action for Gay Men's Health and Rights from Glaxo Smith Kline for a research project on knowledge of and attitudes toward Hepatitis A&B vaccination among gay and bisexual men and transgender people in the United States and Mexico. Sean Cahill is the Principal Investigator of this project. S.R. Cahill is on the Patient Advocate Steering Committee for Prostate Cancer Clinical Trials for Janssen Global Services representing gay and bisexual men and transgender women. None of these activities is related to the material discussed in this manuscript.

REFERENCES

1. Human Rights Campaign staff. ICYMI: New data shows support for LGBTQ+ rights reaches highest rates ever recorded. 2023. Available at: https://www.hrc.org/press-releases/icymi-new-data-shows-support-for-lgbtq-rights-reaches-highest-rates-ever-recorded Accessed August 24, 2023.
2. Wang T, Geffen S, Cahill S. The current wave of anti-LGBT legislation: historical context and implications for LGBT health. Boston: The Fenway Institute; 2016.

Available at: https://fenwayhealth.org/wp-content/uploads/The-Fenway-Institute-Religious-Exemption-Brief-June-2016.pdf. Accessed August 28, 2023.

3. Medina C, Mahowald L. Discrimination and barriers to well-being: the state of the LGBTQI+ community in 2022. Center for American Progress; 2023. Available at: https://www.americanprogress.org/article/discrimination-and-barriers-to-well-boing-tho-otato-of-tho-lgbtqi-oommunity-in-2022/. Accessed August 00, 2023.
4. Gruberg S, Mahowald L, Halpin J. The state of the LGBTQ community in 2020. A national public opinion study. Washington, DC: Center for American Progress; 2020. Available at: https://www.americanprogress.org/issues/lgbtq-rights/reports/2020/10/06/491052/state-lgbtq-community-2020/. Accessed August 28, 2023.
5. Ahmed Mirza, Shabab, Rooney Caitlin. Discrimination prevents LGBTQ people from accessing health care. Washington, DC: Center for American Progress; 2018. Available at: https://www.americanprogress.org/article/discrimination-prevents-lgbtq-people-accessing-health-care/. Accessed August 28, 2023.
6. Beach LB, Elasy TA, Gonzales G. Prevalence of self-reported diabetes by sexual orientation: results from the 2014 behavioral Risk factor surveillance system. LGBT Health 2018 Feb/Mar;5(2):121–30.
7. Caceres BA, Makarem N, Hickey KT, et al. Cardiovascular disease disparities in sexual minority adults: an examination of the behavioral Risk factor surveillance system (2014-2016). Am J Health Promot 2019 May;33(4):576–85.
8. Caceres BA, Jackman KB, Edmondson D, et al. Assessing gender identity differences in cardiovascular disease in US adults: an analysis of data from the 2014-2017 BRFSS. J Behav Med 2020 Apr;43(2):329–38.
9. Chandra M, Hertel M, Cahill S, et al. Prevalence of self-reported kidney disease in older adults by sexual orientation: behavioral Risk factor surveillance system analysis (2014-2019). J Am Soc Nephrol 2023;34(4):682–93.
10. Cahill SR. Legal and policy issues for LGBT patients with cancer or at elevated Risk of cancer. Semin Oncol Nurs 2018 Feb;34(1):90–8.
11. Centers for Disease Control and Prevention. HIV and Gay and Bisexual Men. Fact Sheet. Updated September 2021. https://www.cdc.gov/hiv/pdf/group/msm/cdc-hiv-msm.pdf.
12. Becasen JS, Denard CL, Mullins MM, et al. Estimating the prevalence of HIV and sexual behaviors among the us transgender population: a systematic review and meta-analysis, 2006-2017. Am J Public Health 2019;109(1):e1–8.
13. Cahill S, Miller AS, Keuroghlian AS. Sexual and gender minority health equity in the biden administration. JAMA Health Forum 2022;3(2):e214868.
14. Supreme Court of the United States. Bostock v. Clayton County, Georgia. Certiorari to the United States Court of Appeals for The Eleventh Circuit. No. 17–1618. June 15, 2020. Available at https://www.supremecourt.gov/opinions/19pdf/17-1618_hfci.pdf Accessed August 28, 2023.
15. U.S. Department of Health and Human Services (HHS). HHS Press Office. HHS Announces Prohibition on Sex Discrimination Includes Discrimination on the Basis of Sexual Orientation and Gender Identity. May 10, 2021. https://www.hhs.gov/about/news/2021/05/10/hhs-announces-prohibition-sex-discrimination-includes-discrimination-basis-sexual-orientation-gender-identity.html Accessed September 28, 2021.
16. U.S. Department of Health and Human Services. Nondiscrimination in Health Programs and Activities: Department of Health and Human Services proposed rule entitled "Nondiscrimination in Health Programs and Activities," RIN 0945-AA17; Section

1557 of the Affordable Care Act (ACA). Available at https://www.regulations.gov/commenton/HHS-OS-2022-0012-0001 Accessed October 3, 2022.
17. U.S. Department of Health and Human Services. Nondiscrimination in health programs and activities. Federal Register. May 18, 2016. https://www.federalregister.gov/articles/2016/05/18/2016-11458/nondiscrimination-in-healthprograms-and-activities Cited in Wang T, Kelman E, Cahill S (2016, September). What the new Affordable Care Act nondiscrimination rule means for providers and LGBT patients. Boston: The Fenway Institute. Accessed September 2, 2023.
18. Cahill S, Pettus M. Trump-Pence Administration policies undermine LGBTQ health equity. Boston: The Fenway Institute; 2020. Available at: https://fenwayhealth.org/policy-briefs/trump-pence-administration-policies-undermine-lgbtq-health-equity/. Accessed September 3, 2023.
19. Ollstein AM. Texas judge strikes down free HIV drugs, cancer screenings under Obamacare. Politico 2023. Available at: https://www.politico.com/news/2023/03/30/texas-judge-obamacare-00089641. Accessed September 3, 2023.
20. Cahill S, Wang T, Geffen S. Executive branch actions promoting religious refusal threaten LGBT health care access. Boston: The Fenway Institute; 2017. Available at: https://fenwayhealth.org/wp-content/uploads/The-Fenway-Institute-Religious-Refusal-Laws-Policy-Brief.pdf. Accessed August 30, 2023.
21. NeJaime D, Siegel RB. Conscience wars: complicity-based conscience claims in religion and politics. Yale Law J 2015;124:2516–91.
22. Greenberg D, Beyer E, Naile M, et al. Americans show broad support for LGBT nondiscrimination protections. PRRI; 2019. https://www.prri.org/research/americans-support-protections-lgbt-people/.
23. Movement Advancement Project. Nondiscrimination laws. Available at: https://www.lgbtmap.org/equality-maps/non_discrimination_laws Accessed September 7, 2023.
24. Movement Advancement Project. Bans on best practice medical care for transgender youth. Available at https://www.lgbtmap.org/equality-maps/healthcare/youth_medical_care_bans Accessed September 7, 2023.
25. Ghorayshi A. Many states are trying to restrict gender treatments for adults, too. New York Times; 2023. Available at. https://www.nytimes.com/2023/04/22/health/transgender-adults-treatment-bans.html.
26. Badget L, Choi S, Wilson B. LGBT Poverty in the United States: a study of differences between sexual orientation and gender identity groups. UCLA School of Law: The Williams Institute; 2019. Available at: https://williamsinstitute.law.ucla.edu/publications/lgbt-poverty-us/. Accessed January 11, 2022.
27. Wilson BDM, Bouton LJA, Badgett MVL, et al. LGBT poverty in the United States: trends at the onset of COVID-19. UCLA School of Law: The Williams Institute; 2023. https://williamsinstitute.law.ucla.edu/wp-content/uploads/LGBT-Poverty-COVID-Feb-2023.pdf. Accessed September 4, 2022.
28. File T, Marshall J. Household Pulse survey shows LGBT adults more likely to report living in households with food and economic insecurity than non-LGBT respondents. U.S: Census Bureau; 2021. Available at: https://www.census.gov/library/stories/2021/08/lgbt-community-harder-hit-by-economic-impact-of-pandemic.html. Accessed September 7, 2023.
29. Cahill S. LGBT Aging 2025: Strategies for Achieving a Healthy and Thriving LGBT Older Adult Community in Massachusetts. Boston: The Fenway Institute, LGBT Aging Project. Available at https://fenwayhealth.org/wp-content/uploads/LGBT-Aging-2025-Report-December-2020.pdf Accessed September 4, 2023.

30. Lunn MR, Cui W, Zack MM, et al. Sociodemographic characteristics and health outcomes among lesbian, gay, and bisexual U.S. Adults using healthy people 2020 leading health indicators. LGBT Health 2017;4(4):283–94.
31. Artiga S, Hill L, Orgera K, et al. Health coverage by race and ethnicity, 2010-2019. Kaiser Family Foundation; 2021. https://www.kff.org/racial-equity-and-health-policy/issue-brief/health-coverage-by-race-and-ethnicity/.
32. Karpman M, Skopec L, Long S. "QuickTake: uninsurance rate nearly halved for lesbian, gay, and bisexual adults since mid-2013." health reform monitoring survey. April 2015. Cited in N Hsieh, ruther M. "Despite increased insurance coverage, nonwhite sexual minorities still experience disparities in access to care.". Health Affairs 2017;36(10):1786–94. Available at: https://www.healthaffairs.org/action/showCitFormats?doi=10.1377%2Fhlthaff.2017.0455. Accessed September 8, 2023.
33. AIDS.gov. "The Affordable Care Act and HIV/AIDS." Available at: http://www.aids.gov/federal-resources/policies/health-care-reform. Accessed January 31, 2013.
34. CDC/KFF analysis of MMP, 2012 and 2014. Cited in Belluz J (2017, February 15. Why Obamacare repeal would be devastating to people with HIV. Vox. Available at https://www.vox.com/2017/2/8/14532310/obamacare-aca-repeal-hiv-aids Accessed September 10, 2023.
35. Dawson L, Kates J, Roberts T, et al. Medicaid and people with HIV. Washington, DC: Kaiser Family Foundation; 2023. https://www.kff.org/hivaids/issue-brief/medicaid-and-people-with-hiv/. Accessed September 10, 2023.
36. National LGBTQIA+ Health Education Center. Available at https://www.lgbtqiahealtheducation.org/Accessed September 10, 2023.
37. National Association of Community Health Centers. About NACHC's Work. Available at https://www.nachc.org/about-nachc/our-work/#:~:text=NACHC%20works%20with%20a%20wide,14%2C000%20communities%20across%20the%20country. Accessed September 10, 2023.
38. Liu M, King D, Mayer KH, et al. Sexual orientation and gender identity data completeness at US federally qualified health centers, 2020 and 2021. Am J Public Health 2023;113(8):883–92.
39. Cahill SR, Baker K, Deutsch MB, et al. Inclusion of sexual orientation and gender identity in stage 3 meaningful use Guidelines: a huge step Forward for LGBT health. LGBT Health 2016;3(2):100–2.
40. Fenway Health. Public comment re: Draft United States Core Data for Interoperability (USCDI) v2 https://fenwayhealth.org/wp-content/uploads/USCDI_Fenway_Comment_V2_041521.pdf Accessed September 11, 2023.
41. Scheer JR, Pachankis JE. Psychosocial syndemic risks surrounding physical health conditions among sexual and gender minority individuals. LGBT Health 2019;6(8):377–85.
42. Kim HJ, Fredriksen-Goldsen KI. Living arrangement and loneliness among lesbian, gay, and bisexual older adults. Gerontol 2016;56(3):548–58.
43. Yarns BC, Abrams JM, Meeks TW, et al. The mental health of older LGBT adults. Curr Psychiatr Rep 2016;18(6):60.
44. Grov C, Golub SA, Parsons JT, et al. Loneliness and HIV-related stigma explain depression among older HIV-positive adults. AIDS Care 2010;22(5):630–9.
45. Matsumoto S, Yamaoka K, Takahashi K, et al. Social support as a key protective factor against depression in HIV-infected patients: report from large HIV clinics in hanoi, vietnam. Sci Rep 2017;7:15489.

46. Brennan-Ing M, Seidel L, Larson B, et al. Social care networks and older LGBT adults: challenges for the future. J Homosex 2014;61(1):21–52.
47. Cahill S. Community resources and government services for LGBT older adults and their families. In: Orel N, Fruhauf C, editors. The lives of LGBT older adults: understanding challenges and resilience. Washington, DC: Am. Psychol. Assoc.; 2014. p. 141–70.
48. Cahill S, Valadéz R. Growing older with HIV/AIDS: new public health challenges. Am J Public Health 2013 Mar;103(3):e7–15.
49. Bromberg DJ, Paltiel AD, Busch SH, et al. Has depression surpassed HIV as a burden to gay and bisexual men's health in the United States? A comparative modeling study. Soc Psychiatr Psychiatr Epidemiol 2021;56(2):273–82.
50. Laurence B, Mncube-Barnes FM, Laurence SS, et al. Depression and the likelihood of hospital admission from the emergency department among older patients with HIV. J Health Care Poor Underserved 2019;30(1):131–42.
51. Marshall A, Cahill S. Barriers and opportunities for the mental health of LGBT older adults and older people living with HIV: a systematic literature review. Aging Ment Health 2022;26(9):1845–54.
52. Fredriksen-Goldsen KI, Kim HJ, Shiu C, et al. Successful aging among LGBT older adults: physical and mental health-related quality of life by age group. Gerontol 2015;55(1):154–68.
53. Cahill S, The Fenway Institute. Testimony in support of (H.636/S.365) an Act relative to LGBT and HIV positive seniors in the Commonwealth. Massachusetts State Legislature Joint Committee on Elder Affairs; 2023.
54. Administration for Community Living, U.S. Department of Health and Human Services. June 16, 2023. Older Americans Act: Grants to State and Community Programs on Aging; Grants to Indian Tribes for Support and Nutrition Services; Grants for Supportive and Nutritional Services to Older Hawaiian Natives; and Allotments for Vulnerable Elder Rights Protection Activities. A Proposed Rule by the Community Living Administration on 06/16/2023. Available at https://www.federalregister.gov/documents/2023/06/16/2023-12829/older-americans-act-grants-to-state-and-community-programs-on-aging-grants-to-indian-tribes-for Accessed September 16, 2023.
55. Stein GL, Beckerman NL, Sherman PA. Lesbian and gay elders and long-term care: identifying the unique psychosocial perspectives and challenges. J Gerontol Soc Work 2010;53(5):421–35.
56. Cahill S, The Fenway Institute. Testimony in support of (S.405/H.752) an Act relative to Massachusetts home care eligibility. Massachusetts State Legislature Joint Committee on Elder Affairs; 2023.
57. Bowers L. New law requires training to prevent LGBT discrimination in assisted living. McKnight Senior Living 2018;. https://www.mcknightsseniorliving.com/home/news/new-law-requires-training-to-prevent-lgbt-discrimination-in-assisted-living/. Accessed September 16, 2023.
58. Cahill S, Krinsky L, Richgels C. Fenway Health. Testimony in support of H.637 and S.381, an Act establishing an LGBTQI long-term care facility bill of rights. Massachusetts Legislature, Joint Committee on Elder Affairs; 2023.
59. Krinsky L, Cahill SR. Advancing LGBT elder policy and support services: the Massachusetts model. LGBT Health 2017;4(6):394–7.

Printed and bound by CPI Group (UK) Ltd, Croydon, CR0 4YY

03/10/2024

01040473-0016